THE PARKINSON'S PATH

Your Guide to Finding Hope, Happiness, and Meaning on Your Journey with Parkinson's Disease

LIANNA MARIE

Live Fully Publishing | Mukilteo, Washington

Library of Congress Control Number: 2025925535

ISBNs:
978-0-9980781-5-1 (Kindle eBook)
978-0-9980781-7-5 (Paperback)
978-0-9980781-6-8 (ePub)
978-0-9980781-4-4 (Hardback)

Cover Design and Interior Formatting by 100Covers.

For the people who keep showing up on the Path—the families, the friends, the care partners, and the ones living with Parkinson's. ***Keep on walking.***

Contents

Why This Book?

WOULD YOU BELIEVE WE HUMANS can feel 34,000 emotions? I heard that in a webinar on communication and nearly spit out my coffee. When the speaker asked us to guess, my number—about eighty, thanks to Brené Brown's *Atlas of the Heart*—was the highest.

We weren't even close.

That big number comes from psychologist Robert Plutchik. He talked about thousands of distinct emotions and eight core ones: joy, trust, fear, surprise, sadness, anticipation, anger, and disgust. He also created a "Wheel of Emotions," which is a handy way to make sense of what we feel.

So, why this book? Because Parkinson's is *emotional.* It took me more than five years to write these chapters, not because I ran out of words, but because emotions take time to face and sort through.

Parkinson's Disease (PD) doesn't just affect the person diagnosed—it changes life for everyone who loves them. When you live with Parkinson's, your family does, too.

I was sixteen when Parkinson's entered my world. If you've read my other books, you already know my mom, Val. If you haven't, here's the short version: She was a mom of four, a grandmother, an aunt, a sister, a wife, and a friend. She was fun, generous, witty, goofy, caring, and resilient. She stayed all of those things while living with Parkinson's for nearly thirty years.

Mom met each new stage with courage. Two decades in, dementia joined the party, and the last eight years were especially emotional for her and all her loved ones.

People call Parkinson's a "snowflake disease" because it shows up differently in each person. I agree—and I also think there's a common thread that connects us all: the emotions.

In conversations with people with Parkinson's (PWPs), care partners, and families, I heard the same feelings over and over. Frustration with how long everything takes. Sadness over the losses. Fear and anxiety about what's ahead. And the quiet question: *Am I crazy for feeling this way?* I asked myself that more than once while caring for Mom.

But it wasn't only hard emotions. At least, not for us. For every low, a high eventually followed. On the tough days, Mom's strength and stubborn determination carried her. When fear crept in, we found ways to manage it. When sadness or loneliness settled in, friends, family, and small joys helped lift it.

I've also met people who say Parkinson's woke something in them: courage they didn't know they had, new interests, deeper gratitude. Those stories aren't rare, and they matter.

Writing this book made me revisit moments I once tucked away. I'm glad I did. Naming the emotions brought healing, and it also reminded me of the joy Mom and I shared along the way.

I hope that, as you read, you'll let yourself feel what you've been avoiding, pick up a few practical tools, and remember you're not alone.

One small note: I use the word "emotions" a lot here. Technically, emotion is the automatic response, and feeling is how we interpret and name it. Since no one calls it a "feeling roller coaster," I stick with "emotions."

If parts of our story resonate, I'd love to hear from you. Maybe we'll swap what's helped and have a laugh—or a cry—together.

There's a quote I've heard from many PWPs that fits wherever you are on this path: "Parkinson's is not the end of your life. It's the beginning of a new one."

—Lianna

How to Use This Book

YOUR PARKINSON'S PATH might be long, or it might be short. I can't predict your route, but I can promise the road will be emotional. This book is here to help you make sense of that.

Start Where You Are

You don't have to read in order. I organized the chapters around the emotions Mom and I experienced most often over the thirty years, grouping them into three sections roughly corresponding to each decade. Emotions aren't linear, so your reading doesn't have to be either. If you're frustrated today, begin there. If you want strength, jump to "determined" or "resilient". Make it yours.

Go At Your Pace

Some chapters are heavier than others. If you're not ready for a topic, skip it for now or take it in small bites. When Mom was first diagnosed, she avoided anything that might scare her. If that's you today, that's okay.

Use the Path Pointers

At the end of every chapter, you'll find simple, practical tips—books, songs, questions to ask, tiny next steps. Many came from my time with Mom, and many came from people with Parkinson's and care partners I've met along the way. Try one idea. Then another.

Read Together When You Can

If you have a care partner, family member, or friend walking with you, invite them in. Compare notes. Circle the ideas that help. The conversations you have about this book may help as much as the book itself.

Make It Your Own

Jot thoughts in the margins, keep a short "what helped today" list, or tuck a sticky note into chapters you want to revisit. Return to sections as life shifts. What feels too heavy now may feel helpful later.

If I missed something you need, I hope another chapter will point you toward it. And if another book serves you better in a season, follow that nudge. This is your path.

The Beginning: Finding Hope

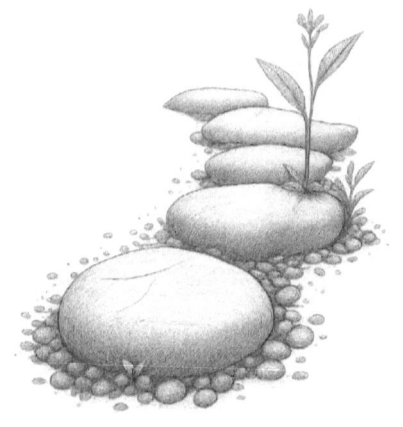

Once you choose hope, anything's possible.

—Christopher Reeve

Shocked

MOM'S LEFT PINKY STARTED TO WIGGLE on its own. The rest of her sat perfectly still. She knew it wasn't nothing, but every time she brought it up, her doctor waved it off as "stress." She tried to believe him; her gut wouldn't let her.

After three years of pushing for answers, she finally got a referral to a neurologist. Then came the words no one forgets: "You have Parkinson's disease."

She was in her forties. In the early nineties, most people pictured Parkinson's as an older man's disease. Mom wasn't the first woman or the first person under fifty to be diagnosed, but it sure felt that way in her world. Even her doctor seemed stunned.

I can't know exactly what ran through her mind, but I have a clue. As I write this, I catch myself watching my own left hand. *Is it in my head?* With Parkinson's on both sides of my family and all the reading I do, it's hard not to wonder. If I sit in that fear too long, it takes over. So, I don't.

When Mom got the diagnosis, I think there was a sliver of relief alongside the shock. "I've got the good kind of Parkinson's," she told me. Her neurologist explained that a resting tremor can sometimes mean a slower progression. We held on to that.

The rest of us were stunned. I was a teenager and hadn't noticed her pinky until she pointed it out. We knew almost nothing about Parkinson's. The only person we could name who had it was Muhammad Ali, and somehow knowing a legend was in the same boat made it feel a tiny bit less terrifying. Mostly, though, we were in the dark.

Today, some people aren't surprised when they're diagnosed; they've suspected it for a while and started bracing. Others are blindsided, chalking symptoms up to stress or aging. Either way, hearing "You have Parkinson's" is heavy. It takes time to absorb.

Shock shows up in many forms: denial, numbness, hypervigilance, or diving headfirst into research and action. There isn't a "right" response, and sometimes it takes months—or even years—for our emotions to catch up with the facts.

Mom landed somewhere in the middle. She wanted to learn, but her life was already chaotic. She was in the thick of a messy divorce and, in her words, didn't have time for Parkinson's.

But illnesses don't wait for a convenient moment. We play the hand we've got.

If you're here right now, whether shaken, foggy, angry, or oddly calm, you're not doing it wrong. Your response is human. And you're not alone.

When shock fades, fear often takes its place. *What does this mean? What happens now?* Let's talk about that fear and find ways to stay steady, even when your mind wants to sprint ahead.

PATH POINTERS➢Shocked

Take a Breath on Purpose

A life-changing diagnosis can freeze you. Give yourself a pause.

Right now: do two rounds of box breathing (inhale 4, hold 4, exhale 4, hold 4) or five slow in–out breaths on a two-minute timer.

Learn at Your Own Pace

When you're ready, start small with one trusted source—then stop.

Try: set a fifteen-minute timer and read a single page/chapter from your national Parkinson's org or a reliable book. Close it when the timer ends.

Notice Your Coping

Shock can look like denial, numbness, over-researching, or checking out.

Quick check-in: make two short lists: "Helps me" and "Drains me." Keep the first list handy.

Be Gentle with Yourself

If you can't name the feelings yet, or your coping is messy, remember compassion > criticism.

Swap the script: trade "I should be handling this better" for "I'm doing the best I can today."

Ask for Help When You're Ready

You don't have to carry this alone.

Send: "Big news. Could use a listening ear. Can we chat?"

Helpful: local/virtual Parkinson's groups (via your national org or hospital social work), a faith leader/counselor/therapist.

Words to Carry

"You don't have to control your thoughts. You just have to stop letting them control you."

—Dan Millman

Afraid

"**Y**OU SHOULD ATTEND A SUPPORT GROUP," Mom's doctor said, trying to offer hope after a diagnosis that felt anything but hopeful.

Well-meaning, yes. Helpful? Not for Mom.

She walked into a room where most people were much further along: many in wheelchairs, many with symptoms she hadn't yet faced. The group wasn't "bad." In a different season, it might have been life-giving. In that moment, it was terrifying.

If only the suggestion had come with context: Find a group that fits your stage.

After that meeting, Mom quietly stepped back from gathering information. "If I'm going to end up like that," she told me, "I don't want to know about it now."

In those early months, fear became a quiet companion. She didn't talk about it much, but when she did, it sounded like what I hear from so many people with Parkinson's and their families:

- Fear that life would be cut short.

- Fear of losing what she loved.

- Fear of losing her job.

- Fear of losing her ability to walk.

- Fear of cognitive decline.

- Fear of becoming a burden.

- Fear of suffering.

One person with Parkinson's told me, "I wasn't afraid of dying; I was afraid of losing myself before I got there." That's the kind of fear that's hard to name but easy to feel.

Early on, it wasn't Parkinson's itself that scared Mom; it was the image of Parkinson's—what it might become. Seeing advanced symptoms up close can be more frightening than the diagnosis.

Fear is universal. Most of us pretend it isn't. We keep it quiet, wanting to look strong, and in the silence, it grows. Michael J. Fox says it well: "Don't spend a lot of time imagining the worst-case scenario. It rarely goes down as you imagine it will, and if by some fluke it does, you will have lived it twice."

If you or someone you love was recently diagnosed, fear has probably already crept in—fear about the future, your relationships, your independence. If you've been living with PD for a while, that fear can shift as you learn what helps. It doesn't disappear; it changes shape.

And let's be honest: Late-night internet searches can spin fear out fast. Suddenly, you're not just afraid; you're stuck.

What helped Mom most was talking, often with her sister, sometimes with a counselor. She also looked for solid answers: She chose one trusted book and brought her questions to her neurologist.

Fear doesn't have to drive. Name it. Say it out loud. Make room for it, then take the next right step.

Next, we'll sit with the emotion that often follows fear: sadness. When the adrenaline eases, the weight of what's changing can settle in. Having language for that helps.

PATH POINTERS➢Afraid

Speak It Out Loud

Fear grows in silence and shrinks when spoken. Say your worries to a friend, therapist, pastor, or a stage-fit support group. Naming it makes it more manageable—and reminds you you're not alone.

Now: send a quick note: "I'm feeling scared about ___. Do you have ten minutes to talk?"

Get Clear with Questions

Fear of the unknown often feels bigger than reality. Ask your neurologist or Parkinson's nurse what's keeping you up at night; clarity calms.

Bring: a one-page visit sheet—top three concerns, current meds + timing, and a goal for the next visit.

Reads: *Feel the Fear and Do It Anyway* by Susan Jeffers; *When Things Fall Apart* by Pema Chödrön.

Tool: a simple health organizer (binder or notes app) to track Q&A and follow-ups.

Pre-Screen Support Groups

A five-minute check can save a tough night.

Ask: typical age/stage mix (YOPD options?), size/length/format, focus (education, sharing, guest speakers, exercise), who facilitates, ground rules, and whether it's okay to observe or leave early.

Script: "Hi [Name], I'm [Your Name], looking for a group that matches where I am. Could you share the stage mix, size, format, and focus? Is it okay to observe first?"

Green flags: clear facilitation, stage-appropriate mix, posted ground rules.

Red flags: no facilitation, "we talk about everything," frequent horror stories without balance.

Alternatives: 1:1 peer match, topic-specific sessions (speech, exercise, DBS), short webinars, or a few counseling visits.

Return to Now

Fear lives in the future; bring yourself back to the present.

Try: the 5–4–3–2–1 grounding: Name five things you see, four you feel, three you hear, two you smell, one you taste.

Option: use Calm or Insight Timer for a three-minute guided reset.

Build a Calm Kit

Have a small "steady-me" kit ready for spikes.

Pack: a mantra card ("Right now I'm safe. One thing at a time."), favorite tea, a soft throw, your current questions list, and one short, steadying chapter (e.g., *Daring Greatly* excerpt).

Place: bedside table or go-bag.

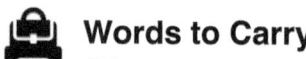 **Words to Carry**

"Courage is resistance to fear, mastery of fear—not absence of it."

—Mark Twain

Sad

MY FRIEND MEGAN WAS RECENTLY DIAGNOSED with Parkinson's. She's in her fifties and, like me, swims with a Masters group where adults train across all four competitive strokes. Sometimes we compete; mostly we show up for the community, the challenge, and the joy of moving our bodies.

Megan is the teammate who never complains, no matter how tough the workout is. She arrives smiling, ready to dive in.

Before the diagnosis, she noticed something felt off. She called it "flatlining" in the water. She couldn't push like she used to. Some might say that's a natural part of aging, but seasoned athletes are deeply in tune with their bodies. When something changes, they know.

Soon after, a tremor in her left hand sent her to a neurologist. She had a hunch it was Parkinson's. Her father was diagnosed much later in life, so she knew the signs.

When she told me, my first instinct was to say, "I'm so sorry." I paused. No one had died, and yet something dear had shifted. I didn't want to project fear onto her future. Instead, I asked how she was feeling.

"Sad," she said.

Her neurologist didn't offer comfort when delivering the news. At the end of the appointment, he simply asked, "So when do you want to see me again? Three months? Six?" Megan teared up. "So he tells me my life has permanently changed for the worse, and I don't get to talk to him about it for months? That's not going to work for me."

I've heard many stories like Megan's, even from well-meaning doctors. My mom, like Megan, felt that sadness too. If you're feeling it now, that makes sense.

Sadness can ride alongside Parkinson's for a long time. What you're sad about may change with the season you're in. Early on, my mom grieved what she might miss, how much care she would need, and whether she'd become a burden. As her daughter, I had my own sadness: *Would she see me get married? Have kids?*

There's a name for this: anticipatory grief. You're mourning possible future losses. I hear it often from spouses and care partners. One woman in her fifties wrote after her husband's diagnosis, "We thought we had decades before health issues." She felt guilty for being so sad because she wasn't the one diagnosed, but she couldn't stop thinking about all they might lose.

Sadness can also come from invisibility. In the early years, Mom sometimes felt like she was lying about having Parkinson's. To the outside world, she looked fine. Maybe you can relate. In slow-progressing or early stages, you may have days when you appear symptom-free. That's a gift and a burden.

People with good intentions say, "You don't look sick." They mean well, but it can sting. You feel like you have to prove you're sick instead of simply living with what you're managing.

Isn't it ironic? Just when you start to accept your reality, you find yourself convincing others it's real.

So, what do you do with sadness?

Begin by reflecting on how you've handled loss in the past. We all do it differently. Some of us lean on therapy, medication, prayer, or meditation. Others need solitude, long walks, or a friend who can sit in silence.

There isn't one right way through. Time helps, but time isn't magic; it's what you do with that time that matters. Let yourself cry. Talk. Reflect. Adjust. Give yourself space to rebuild emotional strength. There is steady ground on the other side, and you don't have to find it alone.

When sadness lingers or you feel misunderstood, it can drift toward anger. We'll talk about that next—and how to work with it.

PATH POINTERS➢Sad

Remember You're Still You

Parkinson's may shape the day, but it doesn't replace your identity. It's okay to feel deeply sad and still claim your humor, gifts, and relationships.

Today: start a "Still Me" list of five things that define you beyond PD. Post it where you'll see it.

Reach Out (Even Briefly)

Sadness pulls you inward; isolation keeps you there. Share how you're feeling with someone who truly gets you—a friend, therapist, faith leader, or a stage-fit group.

Now: send two lines: "I'm having a sad day. Do you have ten minutes to talk?"

If you feel overwhelmed or in crisis (U.S./Canada): call or text 988 for free, confidential support.

Move Your Body to Shift Your Mood

Gentle movement can lighten heaviness and support PD symptoms. Consistency beats intensity; social is a bonus.

Try this: take a ten-minute walk with a neighbor, join a PD-friendly class, or play one of your favorite songs and stretch.

Trust That Feelings Move

This season won't last forever. Emotions ebb and flow as you adapt.

Next step: pick one small thing to look forward to tomorrow (a call, a show, a walk) and put it on your calendar. If your low mood is heavy or lasts for most days for two weeks, talk with your clinician.

Ground Yourself

Quiet rituals help sadness soften. Nature, prayer, journaling, or simple stillness can steady you.

Right now: try a mini forest-bath plus 5–4–3–2–1 grounding (see, feel, hear, smell, taste). If smell/taste are tricky, swap in two slow breaths and one kind word to carry into the day.

Words to Carry

"I am not sad; sadness is on me for a while. Something else will be on me another time."

—Pádraig Ó Tuama

Angry

GROWING UP, I RARELY SAW Mom get angry. Dad was the disciplinarian if one of us four kids stepped out of line. I'm sure Mom felt anger, but she seldom showed it. Even when she caught me in a lie (her cardinal sin), she spoke sternly without raising her voice.

Even when she was frustrated, I felt her disappointment more than her anger. She didn't swear at me, at life, or at the TV.

In the early years after her Parkinson's diagnosis, she hid how she felt even more. I was a teenager, and I think she wanted to protect me.

So the first time she swore in front of me, it stopped me cold. We were trying to book a neurologist appointment, and the earliest availability was a year away.

"That's bullshit," she said.

As swear words go, it's mild. For Mom, it was huge. That one word was a crack in the surface, a sign that Parkinson's was pushing her limits.

Who could blame her? She was coming out of a messy divorce. Her independence was slipping. So much was out of her control.

I've always been uncomfortable with anger—coming from me or toward me. I'm learning. I'm practicing better ways to handle conflict and say the hard things. Still, when the source of your anger is something you can't fix, like Parkinson's, what do you do with it?

You can't yell at Parkinson's and make it stop. And yet, sometimes yelling helps.

So here's your permission slip: If you need to scream "F you, Parkinson's," do it. Let it rip. Sometimes, no other word will do. Parkinson's fucking sucks. There, I said it. If that offends you, I hope you'll stick with me anyway. This book is about honesty.

We're looking for the good in the middle of the hard. Skipping over anger wouldn't serve you or honor the reality of this disease. Parkinson's is maddening. It can rob you of simple pleasures: sipping coffee, replying to an email, buttoning your jeans. It tests your patience at every turn.

In the early years of Mom's diagnosis, weeks or months might pass with no visible anger. But when it came, it came hard. She would snap at one of us without warning or yell at something that seemed trivial. Once, she threw her purse at my aunt. I think it surprised them both.

Looking back, I'm amazed Mom didn't explode more. Some of her triggers:

- Pain that wouldn't let up.

- Doctors who didn't understand Parkinson's.

- Too little time with her neurologist.

- Losing mobility.

- Not knowing what tomorrow's symptoms would bring.

- Being treated as fragile or "less."

- The sheer unfairness of having Parkinson's at all.

And she's not alone. When I attend Parkinson's events, I hear both care partners and people with PD wanting to talk about their anger, but seeming unsure about admitting their feelings. As a daughter and a care partner, I felt it, and I know many others do, too.

So, let's name it. Anger shows up in different ways. For people with Parkinson's, it can look like irritation with daily tasks or grief over losing once-easy abilities. For care partners, it can stem from exhaustion, help-lessness, or mourning the life you had envisioned.

Sometimes anger simmers as irritability. Sometimes it erupts. What matters is recognizing it for what it is: a natural response to an over-whelming, unfair situation. Anger is not a character flaw.

A few reminders to carry with you:

- Anger is human. Feeling it doesn't make you weak.

- Pushing it down won't make it disappear; it leaks out as tension, stress, or resentment.

- There are better outlets. Movement, creativity, therapy, or a trusted friend can help anger move through you rather than get stuck.

- Anger can be fuel. It can help you speak up, fight for better care, and push for change.

- Lead with compassion—for yourself and for others. This road is hard.

Parkinson's may take many things, but it doesn't get to take your humanity. You are allowed to feel, to vent, to rage. When you acknowledge anger, you create space for clarity, strength, and even peace.

When anger runs out of places to go, it can leave a quiet ache: loneliness. But how can we recognize it—and how can we reconnect?

PATH POINTERS ➤ Angry

Let It Out (On Purpose)

Anger needs movement. Don't bottle it up—move it through. Try a pillow yell, a few rounds on a heavy bag, or a Rock Steady Boxing class. Even a ten-minute resistance-band circuit can turn heat into usable energy.

Try now: set a ten-minute timer and do push/pull band rows, wall sits, and seated marches.

Soundtrack: "Roar" (Katy Perry); "Shake It Out" (Florence + The Machine); "I Love It" (Icona Pop).

Cool Your System

When anger simmers, downshift your body first. Use a longer exhale (inhale 4, exhale 6–8), run cool water over wrists, or count backward from 100 by 3 seconds.

If apps help: queue a five- to ten-minute "calm" track on Insight Timer or Headspace.

Turn Anger Into Data

A new angle won't erase anger, but it can loosen its grip. Ask: *"What is this anger pointing to—boundary, rest, clarity, or help?"*

One-step reframe: finish this line and act on it: *"I'm angry because ___; the next right step is ___."*

Read next: *The Dance of Anger* by Harriet Lerner; *Anger: Wisdom for Cooling the Flames* by Thich Nhat Hanh.

Talk Before It Hardens

If anger is straining a relationship, speak early. Lead with impact, not blame.

Simple script: "When ___ happens, I feel ___. I need ___; is there a way we can try ___?"

If it's heavy: ask your primary-care clinician or PD clinic for a therapist referral (brief, skills-based work can help a lot).

Practice Small Forgiveness

Start with yourself. Feeling angry doesn't make you "bad"; it makes you human.

Tonight: write two lines: "Today I forgive myself for ___." "Today I'm proud I ___." Small reps build big relief.

 Words to Carry
"You are not the anger; you are the awareness behind the anger."

—Eckhart Tolle

Lonely

THOUGH BARELY VISIBLE TO ANYONE ELSE, Mom's pinky tremor felt to her like a flashing beacon announcing she was "defective."

She knew it wouldn't affect her work—at least not yet—but the fear of being questioned made her desperate to hide her symptoms from her boss and coworkers.

That urge to hide isn't unusual. Many people with Parkinson's keep it private at first, especially at work, worried their livelihood is at risk.

One of the first hurdles is deciding when to tell. Some share right away; others wait until they can't. Michael J. Fox lived with Parkinson's for years before going public.

The space between diagnosis and disclosure can be very lonely. People pull back, skip plans, and isolate. And even after they tell, loneliness doesn't always lift.

I get why. We talk a lot about the physical symptoms (tremor, stiffness, slowness) because they're obvious. What gets missed is how the disease quietly builds distance, making you feel disconnected from the world around you.

For some, it's as if an invisible wall goes up between the life they had and the life they're figuring out now. Social cues feel off. Conversations take more energy. Easy things now feel awkward.

One person with Parkinson's put it this way: "Before Parkinson's, I loved joking in conversations. Now, keeping up feels like decoding a foreign language. It's like I'm watching a play I don't quite understand anymore."

So people retreat, not because they want to, but because staying connected can be exhausting. Words falter. Gestures feel clumsy. The fear of being misunderstood or pitied is heavy.

That withdrawal feeds a loop. The lonelier you feel, the harder it is to reach out. The more you retreat, the deeper the loneliness grows.

Some find a strange relief in being alone. At home, the guard can drop. No one is watching or judging.

Loneliness isn't unique to Parkinson's. It's everywhere: long work hours, screens, and fewer gathering places. Knowing that doesn't make it easier. What helps is actively building meaningful connections.

It took Mom a while to tell her employer. Ultimately, having a good relationship with her boss made all the difference. He didn't make a big deal of it. He supported her. That kind of acceptance changes everything. Sharing with family and friends helped, too.

For me, loneliness came later in Mom's journey, especially after dementia set in. Our chats became one-sided, and she couldn't offer the comfort and advice I'd always turned to. That ache sits deep.

Of all the emotions, loneliness hits me the hardest.

I'm tempted to say, "You're not alone." Maybe the more honest truth is that you're not alone in feeling alone.

Our minds can tell convincing stories, insisting we're isolated when, in reality, people are within reach. I remind myself of that, and Mom learned it too; it just took time.

There's no quick cure for loneliness with Parkinson's. But small steps matter: a short walk with someone you love, a standing coffee date, a support group that actually fits, a little joy found in nature. To the outside world, these look small. To someone fighting isolation, they can be everything.

Even in the most challenging moments, a quiet determination can carry you forward, helping you reach out, notice small joys, and remember that even when you feel alone, you aren't meant to face this by yourself.

When loneliness is loud, it helps to have a plan for comfort. Let's name the people, practices, and places that steady you.

PATH POINTERS▷Lonely

Lean on Music

Silence can amplify loneliness; music can soften it. Build a "comfort" playlist you can tap without thinking.

Add: "You'll Never Walk Alone" (Josh Groban), "It's OK" (Nightbirde, acoustic), "Lonely People" (America).

Today: add three tracks and pin the playlist where you'll see it first.

Turn Outward (In Small Ways)

Service creates purpose and people. Micro-volunteer if energy is low.

Next step: search "volunteer opportunities near me," pick one that sparks interest, and send a short note: "What does a first shift look like?"

From our circle: supporting Alzheimer's families, expanding access to public pools, and organizing dances at care homes.

Teach Your Circle How to Help

Name what helps (and what doesn't).

Script starter: "Lately I've been feeling more isolated. What helps is ___. What doesn't help is ___. Could you ___?"

Text today: "Quick ask: Could we do a ten-minute check-in this week?"

Be a Joiner (Two Lanes)

One lane for Parkinson's-specific support; one for joy only (book club, choir, pickleball, art). Both matter.

This month: RSVP to one meeting and schedule one purely for fun. If groups feel heavy, try a 1:1 peer match through your PD org.

Keep Therapy in the Toolkit

A therapist familiar with chronic illness can help unpack isolation; ACT (Acceptance and Commitment Therapy) is especially practical.

When you're ready: email one therapist with three lines—why you're reaching out, your availability, and your goal ("I want to feel less alone and rebuild routine.")

Words to Carry

"You made it, after all. You made it, another day ... And you can make it one more."

—Charlotte Eriksson

Comforted

I GET IT: NOT EVERYONE'S A HUG PERSON. Or at least that's what people say. Over the years, I've noticed some folks who claim they're "not huggers" may simply struggle with vulnerability, especially when a hug arrives alongside pain or sadness.

I respect that. I've struggled with hugs in public myself; I call them HIPs (hugs in public).

My mom, though, was a hugger through and through. If she was happy, she wanted a hug. If she was sad, she wanted a hug. And whether you were celebrating or having a hard day, she wanted to hug you, too.

She loved hugs so much that she'd rate my boyfriends by their hugs. A long, heartfelt hug was her seal of approval. To her, it meant they were capable of deep love and commitment—qualities she valued, and so did I.

When I talk to Parkinson's care partners, I often share what I call the Three Knows:

1. Know Parkinson's.

2. Know your loved one.

3. Know yourself.

It's a simple framework that makes life more manageable, whether you're caring for someone with Parkinson's or living with it yourself. "Know Parkinson's" gets most of the attention. The other two often get overlooked.

Doctors help you understand the disease, and that matters. But knowing yourself—your coping style, your triggers, the ways you soothe—matters just as much. And knowing your loved one is how you show up for them in ways that truly help.

For those of us who loved my mom, knowing how much she needed physical affection, especially hugs, was part of knowing her. A hug couldn't take away her pain, but it gave relief. It reminded her she wasn't alone.

Comfort showed up in many ways throughout Mom's Parkinson's journey.

One of her greatest comforts was my aunt—her younger sister, confidant, and steady sounding board. No one could calm Mom's anxiety quite like she could. Her listening presence was Mom's anchor. She didn't try to fix things. She stayed close.

That kind of comfort can't be overstated.

I've come to believe that being present is the most powerful way we can comfort one another. You don't need the right words. You don't need a plan. You just need to be there.

I once read about a simple pain experiment: People were asked to keep a bare foot in ice water for as long as they could. When someone sat nearby and offered encouragement, participants lasted longer. Presence mattered.

Harold Kushner put it beautifully in *When Bad Things Happen to Good People:* "The presence of another caring person doubles the amount of pain a person can endure."

Whether we're grieving a diagnosis, the loss of independence, or the life we once knew, comfort doesn't erase pain. It makes it bearable.

Sometimes comfort is a hug. Sometimes it's a kind word or shared silence. Sometimes it's simply knowing someone is walking beside you.

During the eight years Mom was in long-term care, I leaned on family in new ways. One of her greatest gifts to me was my siblings, especially my younger sister, Tanya. She was a rock: present, reliable, steady. We took turns showing up, and we comforted each other.

Sometimes comfort is a place. For my mom and me, that was the lake. Sitting by the water has always settled me, and I know it did for her, too. Looking out on a still, glassy lake brought us back to ourselves when life with Parkinson's tried to pull us away.

Parkinson's tests you in ways you don't anticipate. It also reveals where your strength lives.

Comfort isn't loud; it's quiet, steady, and real. It reminds you that you're human, and you're held.

From that steadiness, your attention can return to what matters. As comfort takes root, clarity has room to grow. Next, we'll get specific: what to focus on and where to put your energy.

PATH POINTERS ➤ Comforted

Settle Your Body

Comfort often starts in the body. Create small rituals that tell your nervous system, "You're safe here"—a warm bath, a soft throw, a simple, favorite meal, a puzzle at the kitchen table.

Safety note: use a non-slip bath mat and grab bar; test essential oils on a small patch of skin first.

This week: choose one evening to set aside for a "comfort hour" and protect it on your calendar.

Reach Out

Spend time with someone who feels like home—a coffee, a call, or quiet company. Presence is medicine.

Try this: send, "Thinking of you—could we catch up this week?" If you love animals, a pet cuddle or a short visit to a shelter can calm your nerves.

Soothe with Sound

Let sound do the holding: a favorite voice on an audiobook, gentle nature tracks, or one "always works" album.

Right now: cue up one of these staples—"What a Wonderful World" (Louis Armstrong), "Lean on Me" (Bill Withers), "You've Got a Friend" (James Taylor)—or your own comfort classic.

Feed Your Spirit

Let stories make space to breathe. Reach for something that lifts or steadies.

Picks: *The Comfort Book* by Matt Haig, *Tuesdays with Morrie* by Mitch Albom, *Traveling Mercies* by Anne Lamott.

Movie night: *It's a Wonderful Life, Seabiscuit, Field of Dreams, On Golden Pond.*

Plan it: put one title on the calendar and invite someone to join you.

Write It Out

Give your feelings a soft place to land.

Options: keep a bedside journal; note three small comforts from today; write a short letter to yourself or someone you miss.

No-pen option: open your phone's notes, tap the mic, and dictate for one minute about what brought ease today.

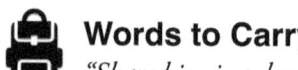 **Words to Carry**
"Shared joy is a double joy; shared sorrow is half a sorrow."

—Swedish proverb

Focused

I HEAR A LOT ABOUT PAIN from people with Parkinson's. It isn't always the first thing they mention, but for many it's a daily reality—and they keep looking for ways to manage it.

For my mom, pain came with the Parkinson's package. She had frequent muscle cramps, especially in her feet. We didn't realize then that it was likely dystonia, a common PD symptom.

One story stuck with me. Mom's toes would cramp in the shower so intensely that she'd have to stop and sit. After enough episodes, we added a shower chair so she didn't have to stand when it happened.

If you think toes are too small to cause that much trouble, you've never had a toe cramp. It can stop everything.

Whenever Mom told me about a new challenge, I wanted to fix it. As a former swim coach, my go-to advice for cramps was to hydrate and stretch. But when pain spikes, your brain short-circuits. It's hard to remember what to do, let alone do it.

So I asked, "What do you do when your toes cramp like that?"

She said, "I look at them and tell the pain to go away."

"Wait, that's it?"

She told me that focusing her eyes and her mind on her toes— and sometimes gently flexing or pointing them—helped. It didn't always make the pain disappear, but it often eased it enough to get through.

It struck me later that what she was really doing was focusing. That simple, clear effort helped her manage something that felt unmanageable, both physically and emotionally.

Focus isn't automatic; it's a skill. Some people seem to have it naturally, but most of us practice. When life piles on, as Parkinson's does, it's easy to shut down. If you can zero in on just one thing, you take the first step forward. Then the next. And the next.

That's what I watched Mom do again and again. She focused on what she could control: movement, food, rest. She tracked how she felt throughout the day, noted her ON and OFF times, and brought that information to her doctor to guide her care.

It reminded me of my training in modern pentathlon. One event was shooting an air pistol at a target ten meters away. The mental drill was to aim for what I wanted ("hit a ten") rather than what I didn't ("don't hit a five"). My husband does the same on the golf course: Aim down the middle, not away from the bunker. That slight shift in language changes outcomes.

Focus gives you something to hold amid the chaos; for Mom, it steadied the moment.

She noticed patterns in how her body responded to meds. She kept logs. She paid attention. When something felt off, she could point to it, which made her feel more in control.

This kind of focus matters in PD because the disease affects both thinking and movement. A major challenge is dual-tasking—doing two things at once, like walking and talking. Most of us take that for granted. For someone with PD, trying to do both can throw off each task, raise fall risk, and make daily life harder. Performance drops not from lack of effort, but from limited bandwidth.

That's why focusing on one thing at a time becomes not just helpful, but necessary. With practice, that focus builds confidence.

Whether easing a cramp, planning a meal, or getting through a rough day, Mom's habit of narrowing her attention and taking small, deliberate steps left her less overwhelmed and more in control.

Focus is the bridge to action. As you practice it, choices start to stack, and with each one, you feel a little more capable. That feeling—having a say in your day—is the start of feeling empowered. We'll go there next.

PATH POINTERS➢Focused

Center Now
When overwhelm creeps in, come back to *this* moment. You don't have to fix everything today.

Try this: when your list starts shouting, pause, inhale for 4, exhale for 6, and say, "One thing at a time. The rest can wait."

Today: set a two-minute timer and practice that breath once.

Single-Task
Multitasking is overrated—especially with Parkinson's, where dual-tasking can be tough. Doing one thing well is a power move.

Next: pick one task, silence notifications, and set a twenty-minute timer. When it ends, stand, sip water, and choose the next single task.

Schedule You
Put yourself on your own calendar. Ten minutes counts: a short walk, a quiet lunch, an eyes-closed reset. This isn't a luxury; it's fuel.

Block it: add one ten-minute slot today and protect it as you would any other appointment.

Set Tiny Goals
Small targets build momentum.

Write three for today (e.g., stretch for five minutes, prep meds, text a friend). Keep weekly and monthly goals simple and visible.

Tools: a sticky on the fridge, habit boxes in a paper planner, or a basic phone reminder.

Feed Your Focus

Choose inputs that steady attention.

Books: *Deep Work* by Cal Newport; *The One Thing* by Gary Keller; *Stillness Is the Key* by Ryan Holiday.

Audio: a focus playlist, brown noise, or Brain.fm to guide attention back when it wanders.

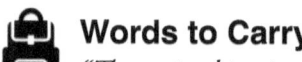 **Words to Carry**

"The main thing is to keep the main thing the main thing."

—Stephen R. Covey

Empowered

AS MOM NEARED THE TEN-YEAR MARK of living with Parkinson's, the disease kept throwing new challenges her way. Symptoms we hadn't even heard of surfaced: freezing of gait, excessive sweating, double vision, and painfully inflamed skin on her lower legs. Some were physically painful; others were emotionally exhausting or downright frustrating. Each one required her to adapt, and she did.

Mom had spent much of her adult life in the background, often in my dad's shadow. Her separation from him, along with those early years navigating Parkinson's on her own, marked a turning point. I remember her telling me she was determined to be independent. That goal became her guidepost.

Looking back, I can see she was redefining herself not just as a single woman, but as a woman with Parkinson's. In some ways, she was shedding old ideas about who she had to be and finally stepping into who she was.

One memory stands out: the day she came home from buying a car, her first big purchase after the divorce. She was grinning, telling me how she negotiated the price down all by herself. No partner, no back-up—just her. She was proud, and so was I.

That win came in the earlier years of Parkinson's, when her symptoms were still manageable. Choosing to believe in herself gave her the strength she would need later to tackle the harder stuff.

She didn't become empowered overnight. It was a slow build, one challenge at a time. Each time she faced a new symptom or a new hurdle—medication changes, therapy tweaks, mobility tools—she worked through it. Every time she found a solution, her confidence grew.

That's the thing about empowerment: It doesn't have to be flashy. Sometimes it looks like opening a pill bottle without help or buttoning your shirt on your own. These "small" wins are anything but small when you're living with a condition that complicates the basics of daily life.

Mom's victories added up over time, like kindling feeding a slow-burning fire. With each success, she grew a little bolder. She spoke up more with doctors. She questioned decisions when they didn't feel right. She trusted her gut.

That shift—from staying quiet to using her voice—was one of the most powerful parts of her transformation.

Before Parkinson's, she might have kept quiet in a doctor's office even if something felt off. Parkinson's taught her to trust what she was feeling, to say it out loud, and to advocate for herself—even when it was uncomfortable. And it wasn't just about medical care; it was about reclaiming her right to be heard.

To anyone newly diagnosed, or walking alongside someone who is: Yes, listen to your doctors. But trust yourself, too. You are the one living in your body. You are the one who knows when something's not right, or when something's working.

I've heard from many people that their neurologist didn't always "get" what they were feeling. That isn't a knock on doctors; it's the reality that they can't see the whole picture in a thirty-minute appointment every few months.

If something isn't sitting right, it's okay to seek a second opinion. Just know that switching providers can come with trade-offs. A doctor who knows your history may offer insight that takes time to build elsewhere. It's about balance, like so much in Parkinson's.

Living with this disease is undeniably hard. It can also reveal strength you didn't know you had. Watching my mom taught me that empowerment doesn't have to look like a big, brave leap. Sometimes it's the quiet decision to keep showing up: Keep trying, keep believing you can figure this out even when you don't have all the answers yet.

Parkinson's may change the shape of your life, but it doesn't get to define it.

The more wins you collect—even the tiniest ones—the more they build on each other. Over time, they create a solid foundation that says, "I can do this. I've done hard things before. I am more capable than I thought."

That's empowerment.

As those wins stack, empowerment matures into something deeper: a grounded, steady strength you can rely on when the path gets rocky. It's time to define what strong looks like and how to grow it.

PATH POINTERS➢Empowered

Trust Your Gut
You know your body best. If something feels off, speak up and act.

Quick habit: keep a simple "PD Snapshot" in your notes app: *What I felt • When • Meds on board • What helped.* Patterns = power at your next visit.

Today: make the note and add one entry.

Bring Backup
If you're not being heard, get a second opinion—and don't go alone. A spouse, care partner, or friend can catch details and ask follow-ups.

Before you go: one page only—top three concerns, current meds + timing, visit goal (e.g., "fewer OFF periods in the morning").

Invite now: "Could you come to my neuro visit on [date] to help take notes?"

Make It a Partnership
Doctors are experts, not mind readers. Collaborate.

Pocket lines: "In my body, this feels like ..." "What options do we have?" "If this were you, what would you try?" "Here's what's realistic for me."

Prep: save these prompts in your phone's favorites for easy access in the exam room.

Celebrate the Small Wins
Parkinson's can shrink the target. Aim smaller, cheer louder.

Try this: keep a "wins" note or jar. *Buttoned the shirt. Walked to the mailbox. Took meds on time.*

Tonight: add one win before bed.

Back Yourself

PD can rattle confidence, but it doesn't define your worth. Skip past vs. present comparisons; own your story now.

Daily cue: post a one-line mantra where you'll see it—"I am capable, adaptable, and worthy."

Set it up: schedule a seven-day reminder titled "Say the line."

Words to Carry

"You may not control all the events that happen to you, but you can decide not to be reduced by them."

—Maya Angelou

Strong

ARMS FLAILING FROM DYSKINESIA. A hand that won't stop trembling. Feet stuck to the floor as if they're glued—even when your brain is shouting, *Move.* A body with Parkinson's does what it wants, when it wants. Some days it's like trying to tame a wild horse; other days you're kicking your heels, begging it to go.

We learned a few ways to calm the wild. The most reliable was exercise. For Mom, it wasn't only about keeping her body moving; it was about staying mentally strong.

As an athlete, I've always felt that link between physical and mental strength. Even when I don't feel like working out, moving my body makes me feel like I can take on the world. It's rarely easy to start, but I've never finished a run or a swim and said, "I wish I hadn't done that."

That's the kind of strength Mom started building, too—not just muscle or stamina, but the resilience that says, *I can do hard things.*

Getting motivated isn't always easy, and apathy can make it tougher with Parkinson's. Sometimes the push comes from people. Mom often found hers when someone offered to walk with her. It reminded her she wasn't in this alone.

Before Parkinson's, Mom didn't have much of a fitness routine. Like many moms of her generation, her energy went to raising kids and keeping the family running. She was always doing things for us, which left little time for herself.

It wasn't until later—after we'd all moved out—that she started prioritizing her health more seriously. And then something wonderful happened: She met Dave.

They found each other at a local dance, before online dating, and fell in love. By the time they got married, Mom was beaming. In the photos from that day, I saw a version of her I hadn't seen before. She wasn't shying from the camera; she was posing for it. She was proud, radiant, and grounded in who she was.

Dave vowed to stand by her in sickness and in health. He supported her daily, especially in those early years. And it wasn't just Dave. The rest of us became part of her team, too.

That team—her cheerleaders—played a big part in her strength. We encouraged her. Walked with her. Listened. Advocated. That support helped her find her own power.

Sometimes the thing that gives you strength isn't what you do; it's who's standing beside you while you do it.

I watched that strength grow in my mom. She stood taller in her convictions. She didn't let others define her or make her feel small. When people treated her as fragile, she pushed back with confidence and clarity.

I needed strength, too, especially as her care needs increased. I found it in my own support system: family, paid caregivers, and dear friends who, even if they hadn't walked this exact path, never made me feel alone.

By the end of Mom's first decade with Parkinson's, the disease hadn't gone easy on her, but she stood tall with it. Maybe not always physically, but emotionally, she was grounded. Focused. Resilient.

Parkinson's tried to shake her. She kept showing up. And that, to me, is what strong really means.

When strength takes root, hope starts to grow, too. Let's talk about hope in Parkinson's.

PATH POINTERS➢Strong

Own Your Life

You are not your diagnosis. Reconnect with the parts of you that don't change—your values, humor, kindness, grit.

Ask yourself: *What do I want to lead with today?*

Mini-move: write a one-line "lead with" intention and stick it where you'll see it.

Turn Up the Volume

Music can flip the switch when strength feels far away.

Build it: start a "Strong" playlist and cue it before tough tasks.

Starter adds: "I Will Survive" (Gloria Gaynor); "Fight Song" (Rachel Platten); "I'm Still Standing" (Elton John).

Tonight: add three songs and pin the playlist to your home screen.

Surround Yourself

Keep close to the people who believe in you—family, a neighbor, someone from a class or group. Support doesn't have to be loud; it just has to be real.

Quick nudge: list three "go-to" names.

Reach out: "Could we catch up for twenty minutes this week? I could use a little pep talk."

Move with Intention

Consistency beats intensity. A short walk, gentle stretch, chair yoga, or a song-long dance break all count.

Try the 10-minute rule: move for ten minutes most days.

PD-smart options: Rock Steady Boxing, Dance for PD, or LSVT BIG-style amplitude work.

Safety: stable footwear, hydration, and support (trekking pole/railing) if balance varies.

Anchor Your Faith (Or Your Grounding Ritual)

If scripture, prayer, or meditation steadies you, lean in. If faith isn't your lane, choose a simple daily ritual.

Simple sequence: two slow breaths → one sentence of gratitude → one clear intention.

Set it: add a five-minute reminder and keep your cue (verse/quote card) where you'll do it.

 ## Words to Carry

"You never know how strong you are until being strong is your only choice."

—Bob Marley (attributed)

Hopeful

HOPE. IT'S A SIMPLE WORD, yet it carries enormous weight. Hope can lift us, shift our mindset, and help us believe there's something good ahead. Without it, life can feel dark, heavy, and directionless.

If you or someone you love has been diagnosed with Parkinson's, hope might feel quiet. You may want to feel hopeful, but can't quite get there. You might wonder what the point is, especially when you're told the condition will worsen over time. That kind of outlook can strip even the strongest person of optimism.

And no one would blame you for feeling hopeless.

Parkinson's brings many unknowns. It's emotionally taxing, and decisions can feel endless. Even choosing hope can feel like work some days. Hope is a choice; only you can decide if it's worth reaching for.

Does it make a difference? Yes.

Dr. Jerome Groopman—hematologist, oncologist, and researcher—writes in *The Anatomy of Hope:* "For all my patients, hope, true hope, has proven as important as any medication I might prescribe or any procedure I perform." That rings true to me because that was my mom.

People often say "Everything happens for a reason" when they're trying to comfort. I've never believed there was a "reason" my mom got Parkinson's. Maybe it was genetics. Maybe environmental factors. Maybe the stress of a toxic divorce. Whatever the cause, the why mattered less than what came next.

Once you're faced with a diagnosis like this, the real questions become: *How do you live with it? How do you move forward?*

That's where hope comes in.

Hope isn't pretending things aren't hard. It's believing there's still something good ahead, even if it's small. It's the quiet push to get up one more time, to try again, to hold on a little longer.

For my mom, hope was an anchor. It didn't always show up in big, obvious ways, but it was there—in the way she kept showing up for herself, in the people who reminded her she wasn't alone, and in her decision to keep looking forward no matter what Parkinson's threw at her.

Her story wasn't easy. The years around her diagnosis were some of the most emotionally devastating of her life. Her marriage was falling apart; the divorce dragged on for a decade. It cost her emotionally, financially, and spiritually. And then, on top of it all, Parkinson's.

It would have been understandable if she had given up. One day, she looked at me and said, "I'm sick and tired of being sick and tired."

That was her turning point—the moment she chose hope.

It didn't make every day easy. Some days she felt strong and optimistic. Other days, new symptoms crushed her momentum. Her OFF times increased. She moved from a cane to a walker, and eventually to a wheelchair.

Hope didn't erase the hard. It gave her something to hold and somewhere to return.

For Mom, people often became her lifeline:

- a stranger helping her to the car,

- a family member planting a garden she could no longer dig,

- a friend encouraging her to start a singing group while her voice was still strong.

Hope came in those moments—sometimes unexpectedly—and reminded her she still mattered, that life still had room for meaning.

People say, "You can't win them all." In sports, a winning record doesn't mean you win every game; it means you win enough to keep going. Parkinson's can be like that. Especially in the early and middle stages, if you can win more days than you lose, you're winning.

I'll talk more about what to do when the losses feel heavier than the wins in later chapters. For now, I'll say this:

If you can face your fears, accept the diagnosis without surrendering to despair, keep learning, reach out, let others in, cry when you need to, and still find the courage to advocate for yourself: You're winning.

And with each win, hope grows stronger.

PATH POINTERS➤Hopeful

Take the H.O.P.E. Quiz

A quick self-check can show where to steady yourself next.

How it works: rate each item **1–5**

(1 = not at all | 5 = absolutely).

Reminder: there's no passing grade, only an honest snapshot. Notice one area to strengthen and one to celebrate.

In life, do you …

H—Hold on, knowing pain is temporary?

> 1   2   3   4   5

O—Stay optimistic, even when the future feels uncertain?

> 1   2   3   4   5

P—Practice acceptance of what you can't control?

> 1   2   3   4   5

E—Enlist help when you need support?

> 1   2   3   4   5

No pen? Record a sixty-second voice note with your four ratings.

Interpret your score (out of 20):

17–20

You're riding a strong current of hope. Keep doing what's working—and consider how you can support others on the journey, too.

13 –16

You've got a healthy foundation. Some days may feel more challenging than others, but your sense of hope remains steady. Keep nurturing it.

9 –12

You're in a tough but honest place. You may be hopeful in some areas and struggling in others—and that's completely normal. Focus on small actions to boost the lower scores.

8 or below

It might feel like hope is out of reach right now. The good news is, you're aware, and awareness is the first step. You don't have to climb the whole mountain at once. Start with one foothold.

Find a Model

Hope is easier to hold when you can see it lived. Your "hope model" might be Michael J. Fox, Jimmy Choi, or a neighbor who keeps showing up.

Next step: save one talk or interview from your model and revisit it on hard days.

Face Forward

You're still living your life. Parkinson's can change the route, not your ability to make meaning.

Cue: write one thing you're looking forward to this week and put it where you'll see it.

Feed Your Hope

Stories and songs can refill your hope tank.

Books: *The Anatomy of Hope by Jerome Groopman; Always Looking Up* by Michael J. Fox.

Films: *STILL: A Michael J. Fox Movie; Patch Adams; The Theory of Everything.*

Songs: "Don't Stop Believin'" (Journey); "Three Little Birds" (Bob Marley); "Here Comes the Sun" (The Beatles).

Build it: create a "Hope" folder/playlist with one pick from each list.

Ground in Spirit

Lean into what gives life meaning—prayer, meditation, nature, music.

Rhythm: five quiet minutes a day. Read, breathe, or sit with the trees.

Today: set a five-minute reminder and place the cue where you'll do it.

Focus On Hope in Action

Real progress is happening; let it steady you.

New options: infusion therapies; gene/stem-cell research; meds for dyskinesia/hallucinations.

More access: expanding MDS clinics; PD nurse specialists.

Stronger support: caregiver resources; growing global awareness.

Every day helps: symptom-tracking apps; stabilizing utensils; smart canes/walkers; adaptive clothing.

Next move: choose one tool or resource to explore this month.

 Words to Carry

"Everything will be okay in the end. If it's not okay, it's not the end."

—Fernando Sabino

The Middle: Finding Happiness

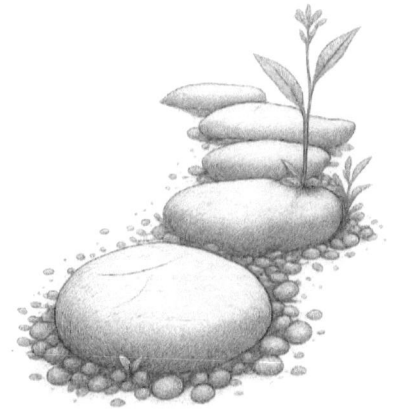

You can't wait until life isn't hard anymore before you decide to be happy.

—Nightbirde, singer-songwriter

Anxious

"**Y**OU WORRY TOO MUCH."

My sister and husband say that more than I'd like to admit. Ironically, I used to say the same to my mom, who was a chronic worrier. I probably inherited the worry gene from her.

In *Atlas of the Heart*, Brené Brown explains that anxiety often triggers two common coping moves: worry or avoidance. Neither works very well. She also distinguishes worry from anxiety: Worry is the thinking part of anxiety. That tracks for me. I'm good at overthinking and stewing, which only fuels more anxiety.

I didn't realize until after Mom passed away that anxiety can also be a non-motor symptom of Parkinson's.

Hers became more pronounced in her second decade with the disease. At first, she worried about typical mom things. Over time, it deepened and changed shape. Some of her persistent fears were:

- Getting stuck during a fire or storm if her feet froze.
- Losing her job as symptoms worsened.
- Losing the ability to knit or play piano.
- Needing a wheelchair.
- Being alone at night.

These weren't irrational. They were grounded in real possibilities. I just didn't yet understand how anxiety shows up in Parkinson's. When she fixated on something, I often brushed it off.

I later learned that anxiety is common in PD, especially during OFF periods when medication is wearing off. If that sounds familiar, talk with your doctor; there are options.

Meanwhile, I carried my own quiet stockpile of worry:

- Not being there when Mom needed me most.

- Dreading "the call" that she had passed.

- Fearing she was suffering, and I didn't know.

- Making the wrong decision on her behalf.

- Losing parts of my own life to meet her needs (and feeling guilty about that).

What did I do with all that worry? I buried it. I numbed it with food, alcohol, and an unhealthy relationship. None of it helped.

Eventually, I realized most of my worries boiled down to one word: control. I wanted to manage every outcome and every future scenario. It took me years to accept that I couldn't.

Letting go of that illusion was challenging and freeing. I still have anxious thoughts, but they don't own me like they used to. If something deserves concern, I acknowledge it. I just don't let it spiral me into paralysis.

That shift—focusing on what is in my control—changed everything. You can't control the progression of Parkinson's (at least not yet). You can control:

- Your people. Share your diagnosis on your terms. Stay close to those who lift you, and step back from those who drain you.

- Your food. What and when you eat can influence how well medications work.

- Your movement. Programs like Rock Steady Boxing, Dance for PD, or Yoga for PD can support mobility and mood. Care partners: Movement helps you, too.

- Your outlook. You choose how you show up, even on hard days. A positive mindset won't cure Parkinson's, but it can make the journey lighter.

Action in the spaces you can influence brings a steadier kind of control—not over the disease, but over your response. That's a peace no diagnosis can take away.

Parkinson's brings plenty of emotional landmines. Anxiety is often the first. As the disease becomes more visible or harder to hide, anxiety can slide into embarrassment—or its heavier cousin, shame. Let's name it and learn how to work with it.

PATH POINTERS➤Anxious

Know the Source

Anxiety can be part of Parkinson's. When dopamine dips—especially during OFF times—mood can wobble. If worry or panic tracks with your dosing, loop in your neurologist; minor timing/med tweaks (plus non-drug supports) can help.

Script starter: "I've noticed spikes of anxiety during OFF periods (~__ minutes before the next dose). What adjustments or supports would you recommend?"

Ask about: dose timing, sleep support, counseling, PD-specific exercise.

Today: capture one line about when anxiety shows up and what helps.

Breathe + Move

When anxiety spikes, anchor your senses, then add a touch of motion.

Orient: name three things you see; feel both feet; say the day and date.

Then move: ten wall push-ups, thirty seconds heel-toe rocking, a slow one-minute march, or a step-touch to one song.

Sticky note: "When anxious → wall push-ups ×10."

Write It Out

Get the swirl out of your head where you can see it.

Try: two columns—*What I can control / What I can't*—or a five-minute brain dump before bed to park worries for the night.

No-pen option: record a sixty-second voice note.

Read next: *Hope and Help for Your Nerves* by Claire Weekes; *When the Body Says No* by Gabor Maté; *The Daily Stoic* by Ryan Holiday and Stephen Hanselman.

Name It

Precise words reduce the grip: is it dread, worry, overwhelm, panic?

Helps: *Atlas of the Heart* by Brené Brown, or an "emotion wheel."

Script: "I notice anxiety is here, and I can still _____." Then do one small, doable thing.

Soothe Your System

Curate what you consume. Limit doomscrolling and add calming inputs.

Boundaries: mute non-urgent alerts; set fifteen-minute app limits for news/social.

Watch: *Inside Out* (and *Inside Out 2*), *A Beautiful Day in the Neighborhood*, *Groundhog Day.*

Listen: "Weightless" (Marconi Union), The Honest Guys (YouTube), ocean/rain playlists.

Calm kit: keep headphones, a soft layer, a simple puzzle, and your "first step" card in one spot.

Words to Carry

"Anxiety does not empty tomorrow of its sorrows, but only empties today of its strength."

—Charles Spurgeon

Ashamed

"Y OU'RE FRAIL."
"You're clumsy."
"You're overreacting."
"You're going to spill that."
"You're going to hurt yourself."
"Do you think you should be doing that?"

People said these things to my mom while she lived with Parkinson's. Some meant well; some didn't. Either way, each comment chipped at her dignity.

I didn't expect shame to show up in Parkinson's, but it did. Back then, I didn't have the language for it. I only knew it felt wrong when people treated Mom as "less than." Later, I learned shame can be a quiet, heavy weight—and one of the hardest emotions to name.

We weren't prepared for the stares, the pity, or the judgments. We weren't prepared for it to come from friends and family, either. But it did.

Shame often grows out of stigma: a negative attitude pinned to a perceived "deficit." For Mom, that "deficit" showed up in her walk, her tremor, her sometimes-frozen face. Those visible signs invited commentary no one asked for.

A relative once suggested Mom shouldn't be making decisions anymore. Another person wondered aloud why she'd come out to eat when she "couldn't even hold a fork." It was painful to watch and hard to answer.

Maybe you've been there. Maybe someone asked if you were drunk when your hand shook. Maybe you spilled a drink and felt every eye turn your way. Maybe work shifted after you shared your diagnosis.

Many people with Parkinson's keep the diagnosis private, fearing they'll be misunderstood or underestimated. Silence can feel safer—but it can also be isolating.

Some women describe feeling less feminine or less able to carry family roles, and that can erode self-image. Shame often wears the mask of embarrassment, but it cuts deeper. It says *you* are the problem, not that you *have* a problem.

I'll admit I felt embarrassed for my mom at times, especially when dementia entered. I flinched when she said something inappropriate or repeated herself. I hated the feeling that I needed to apologize for her. Looking back, my embarrassment had more to do with me. I didn't want to be judged for how I handled things or for how different my mom had become.

Staying in shame—whether you're the one with Parkinson's or the one beside them—breeds loneliness and disconnection.

Over time, Mom accepted herself. She stopped minimizing symptoms. She stepped back from people who made her feel small, even family. She finally stood up to her older brother, who had bullied her for years. That day, she stepped out of shame and into self-respect.

I had to face my own shame, too. It surfaced whenever someone brought up nursing homes. A few friends said they'd "never do that" to a parent—as if I'd made a casual choice over coffee. It took years, but I found the words I needed: "I didn't put my mom in a nursing home. Parkinson's, and later dementia, did."

If you're wrestling with shame, stigma, or embarrassment, hear this: You're not alone. You are not "less than." You are still whole. Still worthy. Still you.

This disease may shake your sense of identity, but it cannot erase your value. And if shame insists on riding along, it's time to show it the door.

When you're doing your best and your body—or the world—won't cooperate, another feeling often rises: frustration. That one's next on our list.

PATH POINTERS➢Ashamed

Spot Triggers

Shame often flares in specific moments—being talked down to, rushed, or sidelined. Name those patterns so you can plan a response (or an exit).

Tool: in your notes app, make a quick log with four fields: *Trigger / Story I'm telling / Body signal / What I'll try next* + an intensity rating (1–10).

Today: jot three recent triggers and one response you'll try next time.

Talk Gently to Yourself

If you wouldn't say it to someone you love, don't say it to yourself. Your self-talk sets your tone.

Swap lines: "I'm a burden." → "I'm learning to ask for help." · "I can't do anything right." → "I can do one thing right now."

Read next: *I Thought It Was Just Me (But It Isn't)* by Brené Brown.

Pocket cue: write one kind line on a sticky note and put it where you'll see it.

Claim Your Voice

Your voice matters—even when it's soft or tired. If someone interrupts or assumes you can't, speak up (in any way that works for you).

Speech support (PD-friendly):

- **Pick your moment:** schedule important conversations during ON times, reduce noise, and face your listener.

- **Say the setup line:** "My voice is soft because of Parkinson's—please give me time to finish."

- **Keep phrases short and slow:** over-articulate consonants; pause to breathe.

- **Bring a helper:** notes app or card with key points; text-to-speech for longer messages; a small voice amplifier in groups.

- **Use therapy:** ask for an SLP referral (programs like LSVT LOUD or SPEAK OUT!; ask about virtual/group maintenance).

- **Coach allies:** "Please maintain eye contact, limit interruptions, and ask me to repeat if needed."

- **Plan ahead:** if calls are hard, send a pre-note: "My voice is soft—please listen for pauses and let me finish."

Quick action: add this script to your phone's favorites:

"Hi—Parkinson's makes my voice soft. I'll speak in short phrases. Please give me a moment to finish, and ask me to repeat if unclear."

Bank Small Credits

Action grows self-respect. Pick one tiny, doable item (water the plants, prep tomorrow's meds, text a friend) and give yourself credit.

Two-line ledger: each night, write "One thing I did" and "How it helped." Read the week's credits on Sunday.

Let Humor In

Life with Parkinson's is serious; you don't always have to be. A shared smile can melt shame.

Light lift: queue one feel-good clip (Jim Gaffigan's *Beyond the Pale*, classic Carol Burnett skits).

Try this: tell one playful line to a trusted friend to break the tension.

 Words to Carry
"Shame cannot survive being spoken and met with empathy."

—Brené Brown

Frustrated

ONE OF THE MOST COMMON FRUSTRATIONS I hear from people with Parkinson's is the invisibility of many symptoms and the misunderstandings that follow. Many look outwardly fine, especially without a noticeable tremor. That creates a gap between how things look and how they feel.

Well-meaning friends and colleagues often told my mom, "You look great," especially in the early years. On the surface, it sounds kind. But when brushing her teeth, buttoning a shirt, or simply keeping her balance took intense focus, it felt isolating. The concentration required for "simple" tasks was exhausting.

Sometimes I secretly wished she'd carry her cane more often, to cue others that walking was work. I even imagined a T-shirt: "Parkinson's: more than meets the eye." PD can be an iceberg—only a sliver shows above the surface.

The result is a stew of expectations: other people's and our own. Friends, coworkers, and even clinicians aren't always attuned to day-to-day realities, so they set the bar in the wrong place. At the same time, many people with Parkinson's set a high bar for themselves, determined to do it all and reluctant to ask for help until they're running on fumes.

Care partners feel it, too. I've met many who try to carry everything alone, worried about being a burden or that arranging help will be too expensive or complicated. But when you keep pushing without support, the pressure doesn't disappear; it builds. The result can be a quiet shutdown or a loud blow-up—both born from overwhelm.

I understand the pull toward independence. You want to do things your way, and you don't want to inconvenience anyone. Wanting help and wanting autonomy can both be true.

There's another layer because Parkinson's affects both thinking and movement. Cognitive symptoms can make once-automatic tasks such as following a recipe, balancing a checkbook, and even keeping up in conversation feel overwhelming. And it's inconsistent. A good day can be followed by one where the gears won't catch. That unpredictability wrecks plans, disrupts routines, and fuels more frustration.

I saw all of this with my mom and with myself. Early on, I blamed her for "driving me crazy," before I learned to sort what was Parkinson's from what was mine to manage. I can't count how many times I stood outside a bathroom door, counting to ten and telling myself to breathe.

Getting dressed took forever when fine motor skills slipped or dyskinesia flared. She loved to shop, so dressing rooms became patience-testing zones for me and for Dave when he took Mom out.

None of us had a playbook. We didn't always handle frustration well. Sometimes we yelled. Then we regrouped and tried again.

Mom's frustrations

- Pouring energy into things that used to be easy

- Typing: dyskinesia sometimes wiped out long emails

- Everything taking longer: dressing, bathing, bathroom trips

- Not being able to plant flowers, her favorite pastime

- Not being able to walk when she wanted to; freezing in public

- Sweating so much she wore a swimsuit around the house (handy at the cottage—straight into the lake)

- Not being able to plan ahead because symptoms fluctuated day to day

My frustrations

- Assuming I knew what Mom needed, then learning—usually through an argument—that my way wasn't okay with her

- Feeling dismissed by parts of her care team and having to fight to be taken seriously

- Waiting for everything: tasks, pharmacies, months-out specialist appointments

- Losing my patience, then feeling guilty when what she needed was kindness and presence
- Watching her suffer and not being able to fix it—the hardest frustration of all

Frustration is inevitable on this path—for the person diagnosed and the one walking beside them. Some days test your patience. Others stretch your resilience. When expectations and reality don't match, frustration is a cue: pause, reset the plan, or ask for help.

And when expectations keep going unmet—when goals slip just out of reach again and again—frustration often settles into a quieter ache: disappointment. Let's go there next.

PATH POINTERS▷Frustrated

Move Your Body

Let your body process what your mind is holding. If there's a Rock Steady Boxing class nearby, great. If not, walk, stretch, dance in the kitchen, or do a gentle yoga flow—just get something moving.

Try this: use the ten-minute rule most days (walk, stretch, or one-song dancing).

Safety: stable footwear, hydrate, and use support (rail/trekking pole) if balance varies.

Today: block ten minutes on your calendar and treat it like any appointment.

Let It Out – Safely

Frustration needs an exit. Pick a release that leaves you lighter, not depleted.

Options: yell a made-up word ("fluffernutter!"), squeeze a stress ball, twist a towel, punch a pillow, or do twenty wall push-ups. A one-page rant in a journal—or a private cry—works, too.

No-pen option: record a sixty-second voice rant, then delete it.

Now: write a sticky note: "When frustrated → [my top release]."

Lower Friction

Small tool swaps save patience and energy.

Try: electric toothbrush; button hook or magnetic shirts; slip-on shoes; voice-to-text; jar opener; reacher/grabber; stabilizing utensils (e.g., Liftware); a timed pillbox.

Next step: pick one upgrade this week and notice the difference.

Reminder: set a five-minute block to order or set it up.

Create to Release

Channel the energy into something you make—writing, sketching, piano, baking, gardening, or photos. Process over perfection.

Cue: set a ten-minute timer and make something messy and small.

Soundtrack: play a calm instrumental/acoustic/lo-fi playlist to steady your system.

Hands-free: dictate a haiku or short note if fine-motor tasks are challenging.

Reset Each Evening

Close the day with a quick check-in: *What spiked my frustration? What was in my control? What's one tweak I'll try tomorrow?* Then let it go.

Read next: *A Small Book About a Big Problem* by Edward T. Welch, offering short, steady steps for cooling anger and frustration.

 Words to Carry
"Have patience with all things, but, first of all with yourself."

—Saint Francis de Sales

Disappointed

THERE WILL ALWAYS BE PEOPLE we love who let us down, often the ones closest to us. Maybe it's because we expect more of them. Maybe it's because they're human.

You'd think knowing someone has Parkinson's would spark empathy from friends and family. It didn't always for my mom.

She told me about the time her brother and sister-in-law called her "frail." She didn't look frail to me. She used a cane or walker now and then, and when her brother amped up her stress, her tremor worsened, but frail she was not.

For years, Mom lived on the wooded property next to theirs, and they often argued over a shared driveway. He wanted trees cut so more cars could park along the road to his cottage; he needed her agreement to proceed. "He wants to make a highway out of cottage country. Over my dead body," she'd say. Seeing her strength wane, he tried to get town approval behind her back. Her own brother.

"Disappointed" barely covers it.

Another hurt: A close friend of more than a decade stopped visiting. The calls slowed, then almost stopped. When Mom asked, the excuses came: "The grandkids ... my hip ..." She was left wondering what she'd done wrong. I suspected the friend was uncomfortable with the changes Parkinson's brought, but I never said that out loud. Losing a friend for no apparent reason is its own grief.

When my older sister was diagnosed with terminal pancreatic cancer, one of the first things she did was cut as much negativity as possible. It turned out to be a powerful therapy, and she lived far longer than expected. I think the same advice helps after a Parkinson's diagnosis: Reduce what drags you down—people, situations, and the endless churn of bad news—so there's room for what lifts you.

My disappointments with Parkinson's are too many to list. It took so much from Mom and, if I'm honest, it took from me too. I was young. I wasn't married, didn't have kids, didn't have a career yet—and Mom needed help. Advice. Care. Sometimes a lot of care. It wasn't her fault, but her growing disability demanded my attention at the expense of my own needs. And that, frankly, sucked.

Here's the reality I needed to face, and you may need to as well: We don't get to do everything we imagined. That's true with or without Parkinson's. There are no guarantees.

Whether it's people who let us down or plans that won't come to pass, we all have to let go of things we'd rather keep. One practice that helps me is to look for the essence of the dream and aim for that. If you wanted to play a sport but can't, could you coach or mentor? If performing isn't possible, could you help organize or teach?

Mom loved knitting and playing the piano. She kept both going as long as she could, a reminder to do what you can when you can. Eventually, the intricate motions of knitting were too complex for hands affected by Parkinson's. Interestingly, she played the piano a few years into her dementia; her fingers moved even when the music no longer made sense.

For many who live a long time with Parkinson's, there's a gradual series of goodbyes to certain abilities and a search for new ways to express yourself. I recently came across a line that fits: "I have made trips before that never achieved their destination but were still filled with experience and laughter."

Letting go can be freeing. It makes space for good things to move in.

We all struggle to let go of what we love. Instead of replaying every loss, try shifting attention to what remains and what's still possible. You can't change what has happened, but you can choose the path you walk from here.

Disappointment can be isolating, but connection is often where healing starts. When disappointment narrows your world, connection widens it. In the next chapter, we'll explore how to build and keep the relationships that lift you.

PATH POINTERS➤Disappointed

Reflect

Disappointment is a natural response to unmet expectations. Name it without judging yourself, then look for patterns.

Try this: list who/what leaves you drained; note when it happens and how you feel after.

No-pen option: record a sixty-second voice note.

Read: Mel Robbins' book *The Let Them Theory*, a simple mindset for releasing control of others' behavior.

This week: circle one situation you'll step back from.

Reframe

A small shift can ease the weight. Use a Loss/Gain grid: For each loss, note one thing gained—empathy, a new interest, a deeper bond.

Tool: two columns: Loss/Gain. One honest line per side.

Read: *Get Out of Your Mind and Into Your Life* by Hayes and Smith, on psychological flexibility.

Nurture: choose one "gain" to grow this week.

Regroup

Refresh your support circle. You deserve relationships that respect your reality and reinforce your strengths.

Action: find one that fits: a PD group, a peer mentor, or a community class.

Script starter: "Could we check in this week for twenty minutes?"

Today: text one person who helps you feel seen.

Redirect

When a door closes, find a nearby window. If an old role no longer fits, try an adjacent version that keeps the spark.

Examples: if piano performance is tough, try teaching basics or music appreciation; if team play is out, try coaching, scorekeeping, or organizing.

Next step: pick one alternative and schedule it within seven days.

Recenter

Return to values that bring peace—through prayer, mindfulness, nature, or quiet reflection.

Hold this:

> "God grant me the serenity to accept the things
> I cannot change, the courage to change the things
> I can, and the wisdom to know the difference."
>
> —*The Serenity Prayer*

Cue: set a daily three-minute "serenity pause."

 Words to Carry

"We must accept finite disappointment, but never lose infinite hope."

—Martin Luther King, Jr.

Connected

"**S**HE'S A GEM," MOM SAID, waving toward her friend and grinning ear to ear.

"What was her name again?" I asked as the woman passed the front window of Stedman's.

"Mickey," Mom said.

I filed the name away, knowing I'd hear more.

I did. Later, Mom told me how Mickey once gave up a full day of work to drive her to an important appointment when no one else could. "She dropped everything for me," Mom marveled. Mickey was already caring for her own ailing mom, yet she still showed up with a smile. Mom couldn't get over it.

Then there was Joan, Mom's confidant and rock. They met at the insurance company and bonded over complicated divorces. After they retired, their friendship only grew deeper—and louder. You could hear their belly laughs from a mile away.

And there were Gloria, Hilde, and Heather, members of Mom's "Gaither Girls Group," named for the Gaither Gospel Band they loved. They sang, laughed, and leaned on one another through good days and hard ones. They didn't know everything about Parkinson's, but they listened and stayed close. Sometimes that's the best gift you can give.

In many ways, these women carried Mom through some of her darkest days.

For most of her journey with Parkinson's, Mom had little contact with others living with the disease. Maybe the first support-group experience turned her off, or maybe life was simply full. I don't remember her seeking out Parkinson's groups early on.

That changed after she and Dave moved to our small-town cottage (population about two thousand). She started saying she wanted to meet others like her.

When she learned there wasn't a local group, she asked, "What if I start one?"

Dave, who volunteered at the radio station, spread the word, and the local paper picked up the story. Before long, a small circle formed: a couple of people with Parkinson's and a few with other chronic illnesses. Their care partners wanted a group, too, and Dave was happy to facilitate it.

Neither group was large. They didn't need to be. Sometimes knowing you aren't alone is enough.

Today, there are far more options—virtual groups, specialized meetups, online communities—yet many people with Parkinson's still feel isolated. This can be especially true for those diagnosed young, juggling family, work, and symptoms at the same time. Finding time for support is its own challenge.

No matter your age or stage, connection matters.

Loneliness is linked with worse symptoms and poorer health outcomes. More broadly, chronic loneliness carries risks on par with other major health factors. The point isn't to scare you; it's to underline how much connection protects us.

If you've been retreating since Parkinson's entered your life, try pushing gently against that isolation. If you're a person with Parkinson's, a loved one, or a care partner, cultivate your relationships. Text a friend. Invite someone for coffee. Join a class or a group that interests you. Keep reaching out, even if some connections fade. Not every friend will stay. New people are out there, too.

You don't have to carry the weight of Parkinson's alone. The more you stay connected, the more resilient—and hopeful—you'll feel.

Sometimes connection leads somewhere unexpected: toward making things again. Let's turn toward the creative spark Parkinson's can't extinguish.

PATH POINTERS ➤ Connected

Reach Out with Intention
Small gestures build real connection.

Try this: text an old friend: "Thinking of you—coffee or a quick call this week?"

Today: schedule one twenty-minute call or coffee.

Bonus: aim for one genuine belly laugh.

Find Your People
Look for a Parkinson's care partner or a hobby group. If nothing fits, it's okay to start small—even two people count.

Action step: contact your national PD org, or search for "Parkinson's support group near me" or an online community of interest.

Today: bookmark one option and add the next meeting to your calendar.

Starter plan: if you're starting your own, choose a time and place, then invite two people.

Keep a Laugh List
Laughter lightens the load.

Watch: *Keeping Up Appearances, Schitt's Creek,* or a Nate Bargatze clip.

Do this: keep a "laugh list" of quick links you can cue fast.

Today: add three items and pin the note on your phone.

Read to Feel Seen (Care Partners Welcome)
Stories normalize what you're facing and offer ideas to try.

Read: *Another Country* by Mary Pipher.

No-pen option: sample an audiobook chapter.

Today: note one idea to test this week.

Treat Connection Like Medicine

Isolation drains hope; connection restores it. Dose it like a habit.

Tool: make a simple "connection plan": Who/How/When.

This week: schedule two touchpoints (call, coffee, class).

Keep it going: set a weekly reminder titled "Reach out."

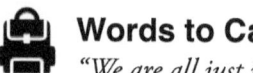 **Words to Carry**
"We are all just walking each other home."

—Ram Dass

Creative

A T THE END OF ONE OF MY CARE TALKS, a woman asked a question I hear more often now: "I cared for my husband with Parkinson's for twenty years, and he recently passed away. What do I do now?"

At first glance, the answer sounds simple: "Do whatever you want—you're free now." Anyone who's been there knows it's more complicated. Your life as a caregiver is over, and in a way, so is your life as a wife. Floating between identities can leave you unmoored and unsure who you are.

A Parkinson's diagnosis can have a similar effect. Parts of your old life slip away. Some dreams need to be released. Versions of yourself have to be grieved.

While writing this book, I came across a Japanese art form called *kintsugi*, in which broken pottery is repaired with lacquer mixed with powdered gold. The cracks aren't hidden; they're honored as part of the object's history and beauty.

That philosophy resonates with me. Good can grow from hard things, and loss can be fertile ground. Whether you live with Parkinson's or love someone who does, creativity is one of the best tools I know for moving through brokenness and rediscovering yourself.

Some researchers have observed that the same dopamine pathways targeted by Parkinson's medications are also involved in motivation and novelty-seeking. It's not universal, but for some people, treatment seems to awaken or increase creative drive. Creativity can emerge in unexpected ways.

In my mom's life, creativity ran before and after Parkinson's. Growing up, I watched her knit constantly—hats, mittens, sweaters for all of us kids. She kept a quiet rhythm: rotate through the children, ask what we wanted, then dive into a new pattern. She rarely knitted for herself, though she treasured one cream sweater she wore for years.

As Parkinson's progressed, she adapted. When fine motor skills faded, she shifted to simpler patterns and chunkier needles. The output changed; the maker didn't.

Music lifted her, too. The piano gave her a way to express emotion and steady her mood. Even as dementia set in, she sat at the keys. The songs weren't coherent anymore, but the act of creating still connected.

After she died, I found hundreds of photos from our family cottage—sunrises on glassy water, fall leaves mirrored on the lake, fresh snow on pines. Parkinson's drew the photographer out of her.

Creativity isn't reserved for people with Parkinson's; it's for all of us. As adults, we often forget the outlets that once brought joy. Making things—words, music, bread, gardens—helps process emotion, rebuild purpose, and find light in dark seasons.

Journaling, scrapbooks, an instrument, seeds in soil, dancing in the kitchen, trying a new recipe—any of it can be transformative. For me, the piano helped me work through grief. Writing helped me name hard feelings. Building memory books with photos of Mom brought a sense of peace, as if I could preserve a little of her.

If you're reading this—whether you're living with Parkinson's or caring for someone who is—start a mental list: What creative practice could you bring back or try for the first time? I don't think you'll regret it. Creating doesn't just feel good; it reminds you you're stronger than you think.

And that strength often settles into resolve. From creativity grows commitment. It's time to talk about what it means to be determined.

PATH POINTERS➤Creative

Start Small, Start Now

Pick one creative thing that excites you—drawing, music, writing, or photography—and give it ten minutes today. If mobility is limited, use adaptive tools.

Try this: set a ten-minute timer and stop while you still want more.

Adapt: fat-grip pens, larger knitting needles, an adaptive keyboard, a phone stylus.

Today: block one ten-minute "studio" slot on your calendar.

Borrow a Spark

Seeing others create with Parkinson's can reignite your own passion. Browse artists and stories, and let their resilience guide you.

Do this: pick one creator, save a piece that moves you, and send it to a friend with one line about why you liked it.

Get Inspired from Home

Feed your imagination with easy inputs.

Listen: an audiobook or podcast about someone who overcame adversity.

Tour: a virtual museum via Google Arts & Culture.

Learn: a short tutorial on a technique you have never tried.

Today: queue one talk, one tour, or one tutorial.

Let Nature Nudge You

Nature is a generous muse. Try a short "noticing" walk, tend a small plant, or snap outdoor photos.

Try this: name five colors, four shapes, three textures, two scents, one small delight.

Keep it simple: take three photos that capture today's light.

Know Why It Helps

Curious about the science? Read a plain-language summary on creativity and mood. You will find that creative engagement often lifts mood, eases anxiety, and adds meaning for people with Parkinson's and for care partners.

Today: save one short article or video that explains this and pin it to your notes.

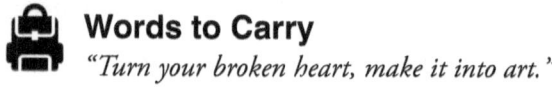 **Words to Carry**

"Turn your broken heart, make it into art."

—Carrie Fisher

Determined

STANDING IN THE MIDDLE of a crowded mall, Mom froze. Her feet locked, and she gave me a look that said it all: *Uh-oh*. Freezing of gait had been showing up more often, especially in tight or busy spaces.

She asked me to help her to the nearest bench, but even those ten feet felt impossible. I held her firmly on her tremor-dominant side, and we inched along. It wasn't graceful. Her upper body tipped forward, and she might have toppled if I hadn't been there. All I could think was: *Don't drop her, Lianna*. We made it.

On the bench, I asked if she was okay. "I just need to rest," she said. Parkinson's had already taught both of us to slow down. I checked the time. Her meds were due. Out came the crackers, the water bottle, the pill case—our standard outing kit. After that day, we added something new: music.

I had a tiny MP3 player in my purse from my runs. I figured a few songs might help her relax while we waited for the meds to kick in. As soon as a fast beat hit her earbuds, she stood and started down the mall.

Music got her moving.

Mom was determined to keep going, and I was determined to help. When music and meds weren't enough, she didn't quit. If she couldn't walk, she crawled. Literally. I noticed bruises on her knees and bought her kneepads. It might sound sad; to us, it was a win. Parkinson's hadn't beaten her.

Her determination also showed up in quiet ways: staying as mobile as she could, taking medications on time, and staying close to the people and activities that made her happy.

I was just as committed—to learn, to support, to make sure she didn't feel alone, and to protect pieces of my own life. The balance was delicate.

Determination doesn't always look heroic. Sometimes it's crawling across the floor. Sometimes it's swallowing pills on schedule. Sometimes it's one foot, then the other, when the ground won't cooperate. Every time you keep going, even when part of you wants to stop, you build a kind of internal proof Parkinson's can't touch.

That same fire is the foundation for what comes next. Determination moves you forward. Resilience helps you recover when things go sideways. Let's build it.

PATH POINTERS ≻ Determined

Move However You Can

If freezing, imbalance, or fatigue hits, crawling isn't giving up; it's adapting. Getting across the room safely is a win.

Safety: practice a "crawl-to-chair" transition when you feel steady; ask a PT for a personalized plan.

Prep: keep kneepads, a yoga mat, and grippy socks within reach.

Today: clear a path and place a sturdy chair so the option is ready.

Train Your Grit

Determination grows with small, consistent reps—one hard thing at a time.

Do this: choose one tiny daily "grit rep": button your shirt, add the last block to a walk, or one extra minute of stretching.

Today: set a repeating reminder titled "Grit rep."

Read: *Grit* by Angela Duckworth, for a quick mental reset.

Borrow Fuel from Others

Seeing someone push through can reignite your own drive.

Watch: Jimmy Choi's short American Ninja Warrior clips or talks.

Try this: save one clip that lifts you and press play before a challenging task.

Build a Start Ritual

Momentum beats motivation. Create a simple cue you can use anywhere.

Options: "5–4–3–2–1, go," shoes by the door, or a two-sentence pep talk: "One step now. The rest can wait."

Today: write your cue on a sticky note and place it where you start your day.

Redefine Success

Struggle isn't failure; progress is showing up, even when it's messy.

Log it: keep a "kept going" note or jar. "Stood up and tried again." "Took meds on time."

Hands-free: record a thirty-second voice memo instead of writing.

This week: read your log on a hard day to see your grit in black and white.

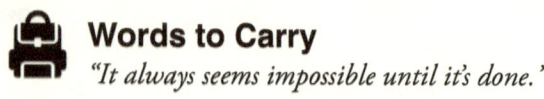 **Words to Carry**
"It always seems impossible until it's done."

—Nelson Mandela

Resilient

I**N THE EARLY DAYS OF ALL ABOUT PARKINSON'S**, we hosted an online forum where people with Parkinson's and care partners could connect—share stories, offer tips, and encourage one another through the ups and downs.

When I told Mom it was live, her eyes lit up. "Can I join?"

"Of course, Mom! It's there for YOU," I laughed.

She needed a username. Without missing a beat, she said, "Keep on Truckin'."

That was Mom. She believed in perseverance. And if you want to live well with Parkinson's, a "Keep on Truckin'" mindset helps.

Mom adapted again and again as Parkinson's evolved. Setbacks came; she kept looking for ways to live fully and find joy.

That ability to rebound has a name: resilience—the capacity to recover from difficulty and adjust to what's next. For anyone living with Parkinson's, or caring for someone who is, it's essential.

Research echoes what I saw firsthand: People who cultivate resilience tend to cope better with chronic illness and report a higher quality of life.

But resilience isn't only about bouncing back. It's also adapting, growing, and finding meaning through hard seasons.

For many with Parkinson's, resilience looks like finding new ways to enjoy life when old routines no longer work. It's getting back up—physically and emotionally—after a fall, a rough night, or a week of OFF times. It's choosing support or counseling when the load feels heavy. It's holding on to joy wherever you can find it.

Care partners need resilience just as much. Often, their own well-being gets buried under the weight of caregiving. That was true for Dave when he cared for Mom. He focused so intently on her needs that he couldn't see what the stress was doing to him—mentally and physically.

Resilience doesn't come naturally to everyone. That's okay. It's a skill you can build.

Palliative-care chaplain Judy Long names a few roadblocks that make resilience harder to access:

- Lack of self-awareness.

- Believing the situation is meaningless or unfair.

- Feeling isolated, as if no one truly understands.

- Believing you're helpless and have no control.

If any of these hit home, don't panic. You can shift:

- Notice your emotions without judgment.

- Reconnect with purpose: What matters most to you now?

- Reach out. Isolation feeds despair; connection restores hope.

- Name what you can control. Even small choices matter.

Another idea that sticks with me is *'mental immunity'*, from *The Book of Joy* by the Dalai Lama and Archbishop Desmond Tutu. Just as the body's immune system protects us physically, mental immunity steadies the mind. It helps you stay centered when life tilts.

We can build this inner steadiness through gratitude, mindfulness, and self-compassion—practices that let us meet hardship with strength rather than collapse.

Resilience doesn't mean you never struggle. It means you keep showing up. You learn, you adjust, and you find a way forward, even when the road is rough. With Parkinson's, that steady return is powerful.

Often, resilience makes room for something quieter but just as strong: reflection. After a storm, you look inward—sifting what matters, what has changed, and who you're becoming. That inner work takes courage. It's where clarity grows. Now, it's time to turn inward.

PATH POINTERS➤Resilient

Take Stock of What's Inside

Resilience starts within. Name what has carried you through hard seasons, then keep those words close.

Try this: list three inner strengths you've shown before (for example: patience, humor, faith).

Keep it visible: snap a photo of the list and set it as your lock screen. Read it before appointments.

Build Mental Immunity

Think of mental immunity as the mind's steadying reflex. Train it with tiny, repeatable reps.

The "3Gs" (one minute):

1. Ground – name one sensation
2. Gratitude – one true thank-you
3. Goodwill – wish someone well

Make it stick: pair the 3Gs with a daily cue such as meds, meals, or doorways.

Mantra: "Fall down seven times, get up eight."

Find Meaning in the Mess

Purpose turns setbacks into fuel. Clarify what matters now, then align one small behavior.

Values → action: pick one value (family, learning, kindness).

Micro-step: "Because I value kindness, today I will text an encouraging note to one person."

Watch: "Helplessness & Hope in Parkinson's with Judy Long" (YouTube) for mindset shifts and practical coping strategies.

Design Your Resilience Circle

Resilience is not solo. Be deliberate about who you lean on—and for what.

Roles: list two listeners, two practical helpers, and one "make-me-laugh" friend.

Bad-day script: "Today is rough. Could you (listen for ten minutes / pick up groceries / send a joke)?"

This week: schedule one touchpoint from the list.

Let Nature Teach You

Nature is a steady teacher. Trees weather storms; rivers curve around stone. Step outside when you can.

Try this: a ten-minute "resilience walk." Notice one example of persistence (a sprout in a crack, a wind-bent tree).

Note it: title a photo "kept going" and save it to a small album you can revisit on hard days.

Words to Carry

"What lies behind us and what lies before us are tiny matters compared to what lies within us."

—Ralph Waldo Emerson

Introspective

LIFE LOOKS DIFFERENT THROUGH PARKINSON'S-COLORED GLASSES. Ask a hundred people living with Parkinson's how life feels, and you'll hear a hundred answers. Some say it's the worst thing that has ever happened to them. Others call it a wake-up that slowed them down or helped them see life in a new light.

Whatever your perspective, it's yours. It may be very different from someone else's, even with a similar diagnosis or timeline. Each journey is unique.

Wherever you find yourself—living with Parkinson's or caring for someone who is—one tool helps almost everyone: reflection.

I didn't always recognize the power of looking inward. Over the years of caring for Mom, I learned that pausing to notice my thoughts and feelings brought understanding, patience, and compassion—not only for her, but also for me.

In the middle stages of her Parkinson's, I often felt frustrated. Buttoning a coat or walking to the car took far longer than it used to. I caught myself rushing her or taking over. I even wished for a wheelchair rather than waiting for her slower steps. I wanted to help, but my impatience stemmed from my discomfort with losing control.

Through self-reflection, I realized my need to control stemmed from overwhelm. The more Mom needed me, the more I tried to manage everything perfectly. Eventually, I learned to step back. I let her try things at her own pace and offered help when she asked. That shift changed things for both of us.

For care partners especially, introspection helps surface what's really driving your reactions: a desire to help that slips into taking over; frustration that hides grief, fear, or exhaustion. Over time, I learned to ask, *What am I really feeling right now?* That question brought clarity and, often, relief.

It wasn't always easy. Mom didn't always ask for help, worried about being a burden. I had to learn how to offer support without overriding her independence. Small things helped. I offered a quiet reminder to step sideways through a doorway when she froze. I framed it as an invitation instead of an instruction.

Introspection also deepens empathy. I spoke with a wife whose husband, living with Parkinson's, rarely left the couch. She asked him to walk each day; he declined, often with irritation. "He's just so lazy now," she said. Gently, I asked why it bothered her. She paused. "I miss how we used to be. We always walked together. Now it feels like he doesn't want to be with me." In that moment, she saw that his withdrawal wasn't about her—it was a symptom. Her frustration softened into compassion.

People living with Parkinson's can benefit from the same approach to looking inward. Reflection can uncover emotional patterns, limiting beliefs, or unspoken grief. It opens a door to a different question: *How can I grow through this?*

When I wrote *Everything You Need to Know About Parkinson's Disease*, I heard a theme again and again: "I don't want to be defined by Parkinson's." Fair. But then—what do you want your life to be about?

Finding purpose can heal. Big questions often surface in significant life shifts: *Why am I here? What matters most now?* They don't need quick answers; exploring them can lead to acceptance, joy, and clarity. As Nietzsche wrote, "If we have our own why in life, we shall get along with almost any how." In hardship, purpose is a lifeline.

Mom found purpose in being a helper. Even when she needed help, she looked for ways to support others. It gave her strength—and meaning.

In Japan, the idea of *ikigai*—a reason for being—is often linked with well-being and longevity. Many in places like Okinawa describe it as protective for mood and meaning. You might wonder, *What if Parkinson's took my purpose?* Purpose can evolve. Maybe you can't do what you used to, but something new can grow in that space.

Psychiatrist David Viscott wrote, "The purpose of life is to discover your gift. The work of life is to develop it. The meaning of life is to give your gift away."

If you're not sure what your purpose is right now, that's okay. Start small. Start with curiosity. And start with the Path Pointers at the end of this chapter.

Often, clarity doesn't come from having all the answers—it comes from asking better questions.

As reflection widens your view, small sources of good come into focus. That's where gratitude begins. We'll explore it in the next chapter.

PATH POINTERS➤Introspective

Name Your Why

Purpose gets clearer when you ask better questions. Let these guideposts help you listen inward:

- What sparks joy now? If an old passion feels out of reach, what's the essence you can still keep?

- What are your gifts? What do people thank you for?

- Where can you make an impact? What moves you (anger, compassion, curiosity)?

- What is still possible? Start with ability, not limitation.

- Who do you want to be today? Legacy starts in the present.

Try this: pick one question each day for five days and write three honest lines. No polishing.

Read for Meaning

Sometimes a good book hands you a mirror.

- *My Little Ikigai Journal,* which includes gentle prompts for what makes life feel worthwhile.

- *Man's Search for Meaning* by Viktor E. Frankl, on choosing our response, even in hardship.

- *The Gifts of Imperfection* by Brené Brown, on living truer, not tougher.

Cue: read one page a night for a week and underline one sentence that lands.

Watch for Perspective

Purpose is often found in small, vivid moments.

Watch: *Soul* (2020)—a warm reminder that meaning can be a leaf, a laugh, a melody.

Today: put it on your watchlist and choose a time to press play.

Listen to Reflect

Music can open doors inside you that words can't.

Build: a five-minute "reflection break" playlist. Sit, breathe, listen.

Add: "The Sound of Silence" (Simon & Garfunkel or Disturbed) and "Carry On" (fun.). One to feel, one to lift.

Create a Reflection Ritual

Make introspection a habit so it shows up when you need it.

Set the scene: same chair, same time, one small cue (light a candle, brew tea).

Three-minute flow:

1. Name one feeling,
2. Note one need,
3. Choose one next step.

Keep it visible: leave a notecard with those three prompts where you sit.

Words to Carry

"When we are no longer able to change a situation, we are challenged to change ourselves."

—Viktor E. Frankl

Grateful

"**I** CRIED BECAUSE I HAD NO SHOES** until I met a man who had no feet."
Helen Keller (borrowing from the poet Saadi Shirazi) has helped
me regain perspective many times. That line reminds me that we can
reframe pain and begin to look outward.

Most of us won't face challenges like Keller's. Still, if you or someone you love is living with Parkinson's, you know long-term struggle and
the sense that life isn't fair.

Let's be honest: When you first get a Parkinson's diagnosis, "gratitude" does not leap to mind. Over time, though, I've met people who—
once the shock had settled—were grateful to finally understand what was
happening. The diagnosis let them act: start treatment, gather support.

Others told me Parkinson's slowed them enough to wake up.
One man said it felt like stepping off a speeding train. For many with
young-onset Parkinson's—juggling work, family, and a chronic condition—the diagnosis forced priorities. In trimming the nonessential, they
focused on what mattered most.

I heard that from people whose disease progressed slowly, too. Years
after diagnosis, some were grateful that things hadn't moved faster. That
was true for my mom. Early on, she faced painful dystonia, her foot
twisting inward so far that she couldn't walk. A physiotherapist fitted a
removable cast; she was grateful to be able to move again.

She wasn't thankful for freezing episodes, but when we learned up-
beat music could snap her out of them, she felt empowered. Dyskinesia
made eating hard, and exhaustion could be overwhelming. With her neurologist, she eventually found a medication balance that brought relief.
Frustrating moments became reasons to be thankful.

When dementia entered the picture, gratitude did not come easily.
Those eight years were some of the hardest. Even then, there were gifts.
We lived more in the moment. And, strangely, because of her memory

loss, Mom did not dwell on deep sadnesses. She did not have to re-experience the loss of her husband or mourn selling the home she loved. Those memories were gone.

Even without words, her spirit endured. She still reached for hugs, lit up at favorite songs, and devoured sardine sandwiches with unmistakable joy. Gratitude did not deny the hard parts; it noticed the joy that still showed up, even in a nursing home, even in dementia.

Looking back on Mom's thirty years with Parkinson's, I see a woman who was strong, determined, and yes, grateful. Even when it was hard, she kept looking for something good in her day.

If you're struggling to feel thankful, I get it. Whether you're living with Parkinson's or caring for someone who is, this may be a rough time. You might be thinking, *What could I possibly be grateful for right now?*

Start small. You're reading this, which means you're still here. That alone is worth honoring.

If you're skeptical that gratitude makes a difference, there's research suggesting it can boost dopamine and serotonin, the same neurotransmitters often disrupted in Parkinson's. These chemicals support mood, motivation, and movement, which makes gratitude a meaningful practice here.

I was reminded of this while listening to an episode of *Chasing Life* with Dr. Sanjay Gupta and guest Christina Costa, a young neuroscience student recovering from a brain tumor. She described how gratitude shows up on brain scans—lighting pathways linked with joy—and how it can lower stress hormones like cortisol.

She also teaches "Three Good Things." Each day, write down (or tell someone) three things you're grateful for—and why. It's small, but powerful. The more we notice what's going well, the less we're swallowed by what isn't.

In that spirit, two short lists—my mom's and mine:

Mom was grateful for family and her husband, Dave. For any day she could move in her garden or dip in the lake. For celebrations that helped her forget Parkinson's for a while. For doctors who truly listened. And for the relief that no one else in our family had the disease.

I was grateful for every time Mom was happy. For the tools and tricks that helped, especially when music worked its magic. For caregivers who showed up when we needed them. For friends who held me in the hard. And for the simple moments when Mom told me she loved me.

Gratitude did not erase the challenges. It gave us something to hold and a reason to keep going.

As we move toward the final chapters of this section, I hope that gratitude helps you find a measure of peace and, in time, a deeper sense of fulfillment in the life you are building now. Gratitude isn't the end of the story; it is the soil in which fulfillment grows. That's what we'll explore next.

PATH POINTERS➤Grateful

Post-It Gratitude

Keep it simple and visible. Write one thing each day on a sticky note—"I got up," "Music helped me unfreeze," "Coffee with Sam"—and place it where you'll see it. Little wins add up.

Today: post seven notes on your fridge or mirror, then read them aloud every Sunday.

Speak Your Thanks

If writing is tough, say it. Use your phone's voice memo or speech-to-text to record one gratitude moment a day. Your words count even when your hands are tired.

Try this: set a 7:00 p.m. reminder called "Say one good thing," and record a ten- to twenty-second note.

Shift Your Lens

Gratitude does not minimize pain; it widens your view. Noticing someone else's need and then responding often softens your own edges.

Do this: offer one small kindness today (a text, a thank-you, a quick favor). Before bed, note how it made you feel.

Make It a Practice

Gratitude is not only for good days. On hard days, thank your body for what it can do, or name one person, memory, or moment that steadies you.

Routine: try "Three Good Things" nightly for one week. Write or speak three specifics and why they mattered.

Widen Perspective

Sometimes, thankfulness grows when you step outside your bubble. A visit, story, or service moment can reset what "enough" looks like.

This month: schedule one hour to volunteer or visit. If you cannot get out, watch a short documentary or read a first-person story and jot down one takeaway you are grateful for.

 Words to Carry
"Wear gratitude like a cloak and it will feed every corner of your life."

—Rumi

Fulfilled

I'VE ALWAYS LOVED LISTS. There's a little magic in seeing a plan on paper and then watching it come to life. Mom was a list-maker, too. On our fridge, you'd find medication reminders and notes about family gatherings, small markers to look forward to. We jot down daily tasks easily; the deeper wishes deserve a list, too.

I recently rewatched *The Bucket List*, which nudged me to revisit my own "big list"—experiences I hope to have before I go. So many people plan for "someday," only to have life intervene first. Parkinson's taught Mom and me that waiting can mean missing out.

Mom never wrote a grand list, but she held intentions and followed through:

- She remarried at fifty-nine.

- She made snow angels with Dave.

- She went tobogganing, as she did as a kid.

- She took a cross-country train ride.

- She saw all four of her children happily married.

Even dementia did not stop her from sharing a Skype moment with me in my wedding dress just before I walked down the aisle.

These weren't epic, but they were ours—specific, joyful, and deeply personal.

My lists have shifted with the seasons:

- Write this book.

- Learn to play "The Entertainer" on the piano.

- Explore the islands of the Pacific Northwest on a Ranger Tug.

- Become a philanthropist, investing in causes that matter.

Crossing things off feels like a deep breath—quiet milestones that whisper, *You're living fully.*

Fulfillment doesn't have to be travel or high adventure. Often it looks smaller and more lasting: reconnecting with an old friend, making amends, seeking peace with someone from your past. These are the kinds of achievements that stay.

If the hope is to reach the end of life at peace—not knowing what comes next, but knowing we lived—then it is wise to begin making peace now.

And while you build your list, remember: Only you have to say yes to it. Your dreams do not require permission. Write them for yourself, breathe life into them, and celebrate each one, no matter how small.

I'd love to hear what's on your list. Maybe we'll even get to celebrate some of those milestones together. Because checking things off isn't only about accomplishment; it's also about cultivating joy along the way.

As you keep saying yes to what matters, happiness has more room to show up. Let's look at what happy can mean next.

PATH POINTERS➤Fulfilled

Live It Now

Choose one thing that makes you feel alive and give it time on your calendar today. Both big adventures and small pleasures count.

This week: pick one joy and schedule a specific time; invite one person to join you.

Share Your Story

Your honest story helps you and someone else. It does not have to be public to matter.

Try this: record a two-minute voice memo titled "My why right now," and text it to one trusted person.

Mark the Moment

Wins deserve rituals. Name what you finished, then celebrate it to build momentum.

Start a ritual: tea on the porch, a sticker on a calendar, or a quick selfie with a one-line caption. Use it today.

Optional listen: "It's a Great Day to Be Alive" (Travis Tritt) as a reminder that today matters.

Learn from Purpose

Hearing how others find meaning can spark your own ideas.

Press play: add one talk on purpose and Parkinson's to your watchlist, watch ten minutes, and jot one takeaway to try.

Starting point: search for Dr. Bradley McDaniels, "Quality of Life, Purpose, and Parkinson's Disease."

Act Now

A dream stays a dream until you move one inch toward it. Progress beats perfect.

Make it real: choose one bucket-list item and write the smallest next step (email, reservation, supply, call). Put it on your calendar this week.

Words to Carry

"Life is not a matter of holding good cards but of playing a poor hand well."

—Robert Louis Stevenson

Happy

OR YEARS, I TRIED TO KEEP a positive outlook about Parkinson's. Inspired by Michael J. Fox—such a beacon for our community—I leaned hopeful in my books and talks. I focused on what could make life easier and highlighted victories.

I thought that's what everyone wanted.

Then an email arrived from the wife of a person with Parkinson's. She'd cared for her husband for more than a decade and suggested I might be sugar-coating things. Her words surprised me. I knew the hardships from my mom and from others I'd met. I never meant to gloss over reality.

Even as Mom faced a terrible illness, she found moments of beauty and connection that sustained her. It wasn't denial; it was searching for hope in a hard place. Still, that email made me pause. Had my focus on the bright spots left too little room for the weight of the struggle? Maybe I hadn't always made space for the full spectrum of emotion this disease brings.

So, I shifted. I began sharing more of the unvarnished truth—how Parkinson's can wear down the body and the spirit, and how scary the future can feel.

Writing this book hasn't been easy. Balancing pain and hope is hard, but necessary. Whether you're living with Parkinson's or caring for someone who is, you're not alone. And it's okay not to feel positive all the time.

When I think of my mom's journey, there were long stretches when "happy" wouldn't have been her word. As symptoms progressed, joy took more effort. But it never became impossible, and that's the heart of this chapter.

Happiness isn't a constant state. Peace of mind may be the more realistic goal. One obstacle is believing happiness is outside our control.

No matter what life hands us—a diagnosis, grief, pain—we still have choices. One of them is how we respond.

Research suggests we can't always change circumstances, but we can shape our attention. We can choose to focus on what remains, not only on what's been lost. We can look for light, even in dark moments.

People who describe themselves as happier often share common threads: resilience, flexibility, connection, kindness, and an ability to be present. These can feel like lofty goals during chronic illness, but even adopting one or two makes a difference.

Being selfless can feel counterintuitive when you're struggling. Yet shifting outward, even for a moment, can lift the heart. I learned that during my own season with depression. A therapist offered a simple mantra: "There's always someone worse off than me." It sounded trite at first, but it helped me reframe my pain and find gratitude again.

Perspective often takes time—and help. Counseling was a gift for my mom in the early days of her diagnosis and divorce. Therapy gave her space to process and tools to keep going.

I know happiness can feel far away when you're in survival mode. How do you feel joy while living with a degenerative illness—or caring for someone who is? Maybe the better question is, *What does happiness mean to me now?*

Maybe it's not a sweeping emotion. Maybe it's a quiet moment, a sense of purpose, a deep breath at the window, or a cup of coffee with someone you love. These moments add up. They matter.

Happiness and health are intertwined. It's easy to wonder, when Parkinson's compromises health, whether happiness is still possible. I think of the Dalai Lama's reminder in *The Art of Happiness*: There's a difference between physical pain and suffering—pain is the sensation; suffering is our response. Pain may try to rob your joy; you don't have to hand it over.

It's not about being happy because of Parkinson's. It's choosing to be happy in spite of it.

Napoleon Hill wrote, "The only thing over which you have complete control is your mental attitude." You will have bad days. Even then, small joys can still find you: a smile from a stranger, a bird outside your window, a warm blanket pulled to your chin.

For my mom, happiness lived in simple things: her home on the lake, time with Dave, laughter around the campfire, grandkids sledding, raspberry upside-down cake, and the call of loons. Those moments didn't vanish; they came less often, so she held them tighter.

She taught me that happiness isn't handed to us; it's cultivated, moment by moment. Even in adversity, joy is there, waiting to be noticed.

So don't give up on happy. It may look different now, but it's still within reach. Let yourself feel everything this journey brings. Cry when you need to, and laugh when joy arrives.

Above all, remember: You're not alone. You belong to a community that understands and cares. Lean on them, let them lift you when needed, and keep looking for the small moments that make life worth living.

PATH POINTERS➢Happy

Ask Yourself

Happiness often begins with a choice. If the answer is "Yes, I want more of it," aim your day that way and allow yourself to become the person who can hold it.

Decide: write one line: *"Today I'm choosing___"* and name one attitude you'll practice.

Define Happiness

Complete the sentence for yourself: *"Happiness is ..."* Your own definition helps you seek what actually brings joy.

Prompt: finish the sentence three different ways and circle the one that feels most true.

Accept Imperfection

Happiness isn't constant; peaceful spells count. Hard minutes don't erase good ones.

Reframe: on a rough day, label it *"a hard day with some good moments,"* then note one.

Try a Laughter Club

Laughter yoga or laughter clubs blend play and intentional laughter to lift mood and reduce stress. Many meet online.

Sample it: search *"laughter yoga near me/online,"* and RSVP for one twenty to thirty-minute session.

Do What Lights You Up

Small pleasures count: a walk, your favorite tea, a quick sketch, five minutes in the garden.

Block it: today, schedule fifteen minutes for one joy and protect it like an appointment.

Rediscover Play

Play = joyful absorption. Revisit something you loved as a kid or try a small, silly adventure.

Try this: list three playful things (sidewalk chalk, an easy Lego build, a gentle e-bike ride). Do one this week.

Build a "Happy" Playlist

Music can nudge mood quickly.

Press play: add three tracks that lift you, such as "Happy" (Pharrell), "Don't Stop Me Now" (Queen), or "Here Comes the Sun" (The Beatles), and play them during a low-energy window.

Read for Perspective

Stories and research can normalize struggle and point to workable habits.

Start small: choose one title and read five pages tonight:

- *The Book of Joy* by the Dalai Lama and Desmond Tutu
- *The Happiness Advantage* by Shawn Achor
- *The How of Happiness* by Sonja Lyubomirsky
- *Happier* by Tal Ben-Shahar

Watch for Uplift (Pick by Mood)

Films that spotlight meaning and resilience can reset your outlook.

- Cozy and low-stress: *Paddington 2, The Princess Bride, Singin' in the Rain, The Hundred-Foot Journey, Akeelah and the Bee.*
- Quiet resilience: *The Peanut Butter Falcon, Hidden Figures, The Intouchables.*
- Joy and wonder: *The Secret Life of Walter Mitty, Marcel the Shell with Shoes On.*
- Real-life warmth: *Won't You Be My Neighbor?, The Biggest Little Farm.*

Pick one: choose a title for the weekend and invite someone to watch.

Practice Savoring (Not Just Gratitude)

Savoring = staying with a good moment for ten to twenty seconds so it "sticks."

Tiny habit: three times today, pause on something pleasant (a warm mug, sunlight, a kind text) and name what feels good.

Share Joy with Others

Connection amplifies happy moments.

Reach out: text one person: *"Small win today: _____. Made me smile."* Ask for theirs.

Be Here Now

Mindfulness helps you notice simple pleasures you might speed past.

Ground it: step outside for one minute; name one thing you see, one thing you hear, and one thing you feel.

Don't Give Up On Happy

Happiness may look different now, but it's still possible, even on hard days.

Gentle reminder: when joy arrives—however small—let yourself feel it without apology.

Words to Carry

"My happiness grows in direct proportion to my acceptance and in inverse proportion to my expectations."

—Michael J. Fox

The End: Finding Meaning

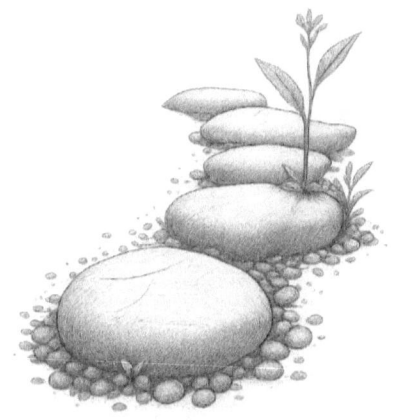

He who has a why to live for can bear with almost any how.

—Friedrich Nietzsche

Brave

NO ONE WARNED US how much courage it would take to live with Parkinson's.

As Mom entered her third decade with the disease, new signs told us the road was steepening: memory slips, longer OFF times, painful dyskinesia, and more frequent hallucinations. They hinted at harder miles ahead.

Before writing this book, I hadn't fully grasped how brave she was in those years. She named me her power of attorney before it was required, a clear-eyed act of courage that acknowledged limits and welcomed help.

I often tried to keep a brave face around her, worried my own fear would add weight to hers. If she wavered, I wanted to be steady. I wasn't always successful. Many days, I feared for her future and wondered how to face my own without her.

Working on this chapter gave me language that helps: Bravery is the quick act in the moment of danger; courage is choosing to act with fear in the room. People with Parkinson's—and the people who love them—need both.

Courage looks like telling someone you've been diagnosed. It looks like facing uncertainty at work. It looks like getting up again on a day when the disease feels relentless.

For me, being brave meant showing up in her later years of long-term care—walking into her room not knowing what state she'd be in, and staying anyway.

Brené Brown reminds us that courage isn't only heroic deeds; it's speaking honestly from the heart and meeting life as it is. Mom did that. Her faith helped. Trust in a God who saw her gave her strength beyond herself.

Bravery also means seeking help for the mind: anxiety, depression, panic. Naming those and asking for support is its own kind of strong.

How Mom showed bravery
- Faced public moments of dyskinesia and freezing without hiding.
- Went to counseling when the emotional toll spiked.
- Spoke honestly with family and friends about hard days.
- Pushed back against stigma and smallness.
- Met each new symptom without knowing what would follow.
- Accepted dementia and, later, the move to long-term care.

How I tried to be brave
- Helped her navigate tough moments even when I felt unsure.
- Let go of the illusion of control over the disease.
- Walked into her care-home room ready for whatever I found.
- Made room for my fear and kept showing up.

What about you? Think back to your own brave moments—large or small—when you showed up without feeling ready. Maybe you spoke up in an appointment, asked for help, or got out of bed on a hard morning. Those acts count. They're proof that courage is already in you, even when fear walks beside it.

And fear does still walk beside it. Even with courage on board, fear circles back. It deserves another look—with new tools and a little more light.

PATH POINTERS ➤ Brave

Build Courage Like a Muscle

Courage grows with small, repeatable reps, not grand gestures.

Try this: choose one moment today to speak up, show up, or stay with discomfort for ten seconds longer.

Track it: make a tiny "brave tally" and add a ✔ to today's calendar when you do it.

Name It, Then Move

Labeling fear loosens its grip, and one tiny action keeps you from stalling.

Script: "I notice fear of ___. I can control ___. Next tiny step: ___."

Now: send one ask, state one need, or take the first physical step.

Rehearse the Hard Part

Brief mental practice builds follow-through when the stakes feel high.

If/then plan: "If I freeze at a doorway, then I'll step sideways, count '1-2-3,' and shift my weight."

This week: write one if/then for a real scenario (clinic question, crowded aisle, hard phone call).

Ask for Backup on Purpose

Requesting help is courageous, not burdensome. Be specific and time-bound.

Micro-asks: "Could you pick up meds Friday at 3 p.m.?" "Will you join Tuesday's visit and take notes?"

Borrow courage: queue one talk or chapter that steadies you (for example, a chapter from *Daring Greatly* by Brené Brown).

Anchor to What Matters

Bravery sticks when it serves your values, and your body is primed to act.

Card it: choose one weekly value ("Steadiness," "Honesty," "Kindness") and glance at it before hard moments.

Press play: add two bold-feeling songs: "Rise Up" (Andra Day); "Brave" (Sara Bareilles), and use them before challenging tasks.

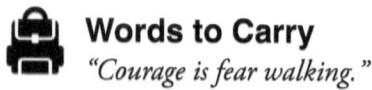 **Words to Carry**
"Courage is fear walking."

—Susan David

Afraid (Part II)

AFTER ONE OF MY CARE TALKS, a woman in her sixties asked, "My husband is afraid of dying from Parkinson's. What should I do?" I often reassure people that many die *with* Parkinson's rather than from it, but her question felt deeper.

Her husband was in the late stages. Canceled trips, lost memories, and shrinking independence had rewritten their retirement. She wasn't only afraid of the end; she was afraid of the road to it.

In the early years, fear often centers on an unknown future. As the disease advances, the fears shift: suffering, loneliness, decline. My mom felt those, too.

As Parkinson's progressed, tension at home grew. Mom and Dave were arguing more often than not, and neither of them was doing well. They agreed to a trial separation, hoping that living apart would give them space to look after their own health and focus on their relationship instead of the disease.

Instead, the fear of living alone, together with her round-the-clock needs, pushed us toward a gut-wrenching decision: long-term care. We chose the first available facility. It was far from family, dreary, and not geared to Parkinson's. We promised it would be temporary, and Mom held on to that.

A few months later, a hospital-based long-term care unit near Dave had a room. We were relieved. Then the visits we'd hoped for didn't happen. Friends had their own health issues, or couldn't face seeing her there. Dave tried, but he was struggling, too. Mom spent more time alone than with people she loved.

Staffing ratios left little time for anything beyond basic care. Outings, hobbies, and simple outside time were rare. It was better than the first place, but it wasn't a fit for Mom's life.

As her power of attorney for care, I felt the pull to fix everything—and the fear of failing her if I didn't. The guilt-fueled anxiety didn't help either of us.

After many difficult conversations, Mom agreed to move closer to my sister and me. We toured options, found a place that felt right, and soon got the call: A room was open. For a moment, we exhaled.

Looking back, we had no idea what was coming. Even with the best intentions, you can lose the map.

Next, we'll talk about that feeling—what it means to be lost, and how to find your footing again.

PATH POINTERS>Afraid (Part II)

Pause on Purpose

When fear revs the engine (often disguised as anger), pause. Breathe slowly and name what you know right now. Clarity first, reaction second.

Set a cue: when you notice a spike, place a hand on your chest and say, "Right now I'm safe. One next step."

Helpful tools: a simple breathing timer (Insight Timer, Calm) or your watch's Breathe function.

Prepare Ahead

Readiness calms the nervous system. If choking is a worry, learn the Heimlich and practice slow, mindful eating. Planning for "what ifs" turns panic into a plan.

Book it: take a basic first-aid, CPR, and choking course; post a one-page "What to do if ..." sheet on the fridge.

Helpful tools: Red Cross First Aid app, medical ID jewelry, and updated emergency contacts on your phone.

Get Your Papers in Order

Facing hard topics is not giving up. A will, power of attorney, and advance directives ease everyone's mind.

Block thirty minutes: schedule a "paperwork session" this week to start or update key documents.

Helpful tools: a simple life-file binder (contacts, meds list, directives), a password manager, and a wallet card with meds and allergies.

Find Your People

Fear grows in isolation. Share what keeps you up at night with someone safe: a friend, support group, counselor, or chaplain. Being heard lightens the load.

Send one text: "Could we talk this week? I'd value a listening ear."

Helpful tools: a short "What I need" note on your phone (rides, a check-in call, prayer) so asking is easier in the moment.

Stack Small Wins

You cannot control every outcome, but you can build confidence one action at a time.

Start a one-line log: each night, jot "Today I handled ___" or "I showed up for ___." Read it back on hard days.

Helpful tools: index cards for mantras ("One thing at a time," "I can handle this minute"); a weekly mini-goal sticky on the fridge.

Words to Carry

"You gain strength, courage and confidence by every experience in which you really stop to look fear in the face ... You must do the thing you think you cannot do."

—Eleanor Roosevelt

Lost

IN HER ESSAY *Effect of Health on Self-Identity: An Autoethnography*, Karla Hildebrandt Kroeker writes:

> I often can't quite tell if I'm picking through the debris left after the bomb of illness exploded in my life, searching for any pieces of my previous self that can be salvaged, or if I'm in the process of raising a new self from the ashes of what came before.

As someone who loved and lived alongside a person with late-stage Parkinson's, dementia in the mix, I recognize that rebuild.

It's obvious to say Parkinson's changes the person who has it. It also changes the care partner.

Twenty-two years in, we sold our beloved cottage to pay for Mom's long-term care. It was more than a place; it was our sanctuary. Losing it, while slowly losing Mom, was one of the hardest things I've lived through. I'm grateful the sale covered her eight years of care, but even after moving her closer to my sister and me, I felt unmoored.

I didn't expect the move to the new home—I'll call it The Pines—to hit Mom so hard. She had already lived in two facilities. I assumed she'd adjust. I underestimated what she was leaving: the town she loved and the man she loved. Despite their ups and downs, she loved Dave deeply. I also underestimated Parkinson's and its new companion, dementia.

Whether it was the stress of the move, disease progression, or both, her decline sped up. She grew angry with me, blamed me for "locking her up," and once called 911 from her room, demanding the police let her out. Those were disorienting days. I had to face the fact that Mom was no longer my parent in the old sense. Our roles had shifted, and fast.

I had little personal experience with dementia, though I remembered my grandfather's Alzheimer's. My aunt, who had cared for him, became my guide. When I called her in tears after Mom scolded me, she said, "Don't take it personally. The people closest to the person with dementia get the worst of it." Oddly, that helped. It meant we were still close, even if her frustration was landing on me.

My aunt also helped me trust my instincts. A head nurse at The Pines told me Mom had an "anger problem" and should be moved to the special behaviors unit. When I asked for examples, the "pattern" came down to one incident: Mom had pushed a male caregiver away. I knew she was confused and still adjusting, but she wasn't an angry person. I said no—more than once. Later, I learned they needed family permission to move residents between units. If I hadn't spoken up, she would have been moved. Within a few months, the outbursts faded, and the subject never came up again.

Over time, I understood what The Pines could and couldn't offer. I also learned that the things my sister and I had prioritized—modern amenities, spotless halls, a fresh smell—weren't the most important. Advocacy was. Being present, asking questions, noticing the small things, and pushing when something felt off became part of my job.

I did find my footing. But the cost was real. The emotion, the decisions, the need to keep showing up—it wore me down.

Let's be honest about that cost next: Exhausted—what it felt like, and how I tried to carry it.

PATH POINTERS>Lost

Ask Those Who've Been There

Big decisions (like long-term care) get lighter when you borrow someone else's hindsight. People who've walked this road offer context outsiders can't.

Action: list three people (friend, social worker, seasoned caregiver).

Book: one twenty-minute call this week.

Bring: three questions—"What worked?" "What would you change?" "What should I watch in month one?"

Trust Your Path

"Parenting a parent" is disorienting. You do not need every answer today.

Pocket card: write two lines and keep them visible: *"I don't have to know everything today. My next right step is __."* Update the blank each morning.

Return to What Steadies You

If faith once grounded you, let it again—even in small doses. If not, choose a quiet practice that brings you back to yourself.

Tiny habit: set a five-minute pause by a daily cue (kettle, coffee maker). Read one short passage or quote, say a simple prayer, or sit in stillness.

Protect Your Basics

When you feel lost, start with anchors: sleep, food, movement, connection. These are not luxuries; they are stability.

This week: choose two non-negotiables (e.g., a ten-minute walk and one real meal, or lights-out by 10 p.m. and one supportive text). Put them on your calendar like appointments.

Find Your Touch Tree

In the woods, the rule is STOP: Stop, Think, Observe, Plan. A Touch Tree is your life anchor you return to when overwhelmed.

Use it: pick one clear anchor (a specific chair + five slow breaths; a one-line prayer; a "return" journal page; a check-in text to one friend).

Set a safe radius: try a fifteen to thirty-minute out-and-back on one task, then return to your anchor and note what changed.

Note: *"Touch Tree" language popularized by Glennon Doyle.*

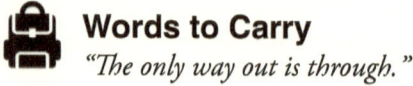 **Words to Carry**
"The only way out is through."

—Robert Frost

Exhausted

SIT IN ON A SUPPORT GROUP for Parkinson's care partners in the late stages, and you'll hear the hard truth. Many describe life as being on call all day and all night. Unlike nurses with shifts, caregivers rarely get a handoff.

For families in the long haul, Parkinson's isn't just tiring; it's draining—physically and emotionally. If you're not careful, it will wear you down.

And if you're living with Parkinson's and reading this, hear me: I'm talking about the disease, not you. You're not draining. The bleeping Parkinson's is.

In Mom's later years, the days were long and demanding. She needed help with almost everything: dressing, bathing, and emotional steadiness. Anxiety, paranoia, and hallucinations could arrive on the same afternoon. She told me she saw spiders on my face, black holes near the grandkids, police on their way, or male staff who might hurt her.

Some of it traced back to medication. Amantadine helped her dyskinesia, yet it also stirred hallucinations. Around the same time, she began nodding off multiple times a day. Insomnia showed up at night. The double hit wrecked her sleep.

Excessive daytime sleepiness is common in Parkinson's. In her case, adjusting meds eased the hallucinations and the daytime dozing. The lingering paranoia we chalked up to dementia and met with reassurance, redirection, and as much calm as we could offer.

Balancing medication became its own job: Find the mix that helps without creating a new problem. And that was only one part of the work.

Caregiving in late-stage Parkinson's is a nonstop operation. You manage meds and appointments, chase answers through a maze of systems, carry the emotional load, and lose sleep. You play nurse, therapist, and advocate—sometimes in the same hour.

If you're exhausted to the core, here's an idea that helped me understand why. In *Burnout*, Emily and Amelia Nagoski write, "Emotions are tunnels. If you go all the way through them, you get to the light at the end." Exhaustion builds when we get stuck halfway.

Recovery asks us to move through, to let grief, fear, or frustration crest and pass, instead of shoving it down. I wish I'd had those words during our first months at The Pines. I spent so much energy outrunning my feelings that I wore myself out more than once.

The truth is, the work doesn't end at home. Sometimes the systems that should help make you even more tired. In the next chapter, we'll talk about what happens when care falls short—and how to recognize and respond to neglect.

PATH POINTERS ≻ Exhausted

Talk to Your Clinician

If sleep is off—insomnia at night or nodding off by day—loop your clinician in. Small timing or dose tweaks, or a sleep study, can help.

Bring: a one-page sleep snapshot (bed/wake times, naps, meds and timing, caffeine, what helps/what hurts, nighttime symptoms like REM behavior).

Ask about: medication adjustments (including amantadine timing), non-drug options, and whether excessive daytime sleepiness is medication-related.

Settle Emotional Fatigue

When you feel wrung out, calm the body first so the mind can follow.

Try now (one to two minutes): a "physiological sigh" (two short inhales through the nose, slow exhale through the mouth), a gentle shake-out of arms and legs, or humming to cue the vagus nerve. Repeat three to five times.

Protect Your Recharge

Rest isn't a reward; it's maintenance.

This week: claim one protected block of sixty to ninety minutes. Arrange coverage via a sibling/friend/faith group/respite. If employed, check your Employee Assistance Program (EAP) or use Paid Time Off (PTO); if retired, call an adult day program to explore options.

Give Yourself Grace

You are human, not a machine. Some days, "good enough" is a win.

Post this where you'll see it: "Today I'm allowed to rest." or "I did what I could with the energy I had."

When guilt pops up, read it aloud once and move on.

Change the Scene
A slight shift can lift the fog.

Today: step outside for ten minutes, sit by a bright window, or call someone you miss.

By the weekend: plan one thirty-minute mini-escape (a park bench, a quiet café, or a drive to the water) and set a reminder now.

Words to Carry
"Courage is not having the strength to go on; it is going on when you don't have the strength."

—Theodore Roosevelt

Neglected

ONE DAY DURING A ROUTINE VISIT to The Pines, I found Mom sitting alone in the hallway outside her room: in her wheelchair, hair a mess, one shoe missing, summer clothes in the middle of winter. Her glasses—her lifeline—were nowhere. My heart sank. She looked like someone who had been forgotten.

To mask my upset, I cracked a joke about the missing shoe. Inside, I felt devastated, as if I had sent the woman who spent her life caring for me into a situation she never would have chosen.

I know dementia care is hard. It really is. And not everyone is cut out for it. But Mom was on a dementia-designated wing, under trained professionals. I expected better.

Another afternoon, I found her in the courtyard on a hot day, face flushed and skin too warm. I rushed her inside and wondered how long she would have been left there. Who checks when no one is visiting?

Looking back, my sister and I misjudged The Pines. It looked good on the surface, but we missed warning signs, such as constant staff turnover. When caregivers are overstretched and underpaid, consistency and genuine care slip.

Within the first year, Mom lost more than thirty pounds. Her doctor called me and said gently that if nothing changed, she might have less than a year, and "she'll most likely starve to death." I hadn't seen her refusing meals; dementia had taken her ability to feed herself.

With low staffing and few volunteers, shortcuts became the norm. The "win-win" became grilled cheese at every meal because she could manage it on her own. As her appetite faded, that shortcut crossed into neglect.

It wasn't awful all the time. Some staff were deeply kind, and on their shifts, I breathed easier. But they often moved on, and too many days fell to worn-down caregivers with little bandwidth left.

I didn't expect anyone to cure Parkinson's or dementia. I wanted compassion. I wanted people to show up with empathy.

At first, I hesitated to speak up. Over time, I found a few nurses I could trust and began advocating harder. Hearing their side helped me understand the constraints. It also made me angrier, because once you see how the system fails people like my mom, it's hard not to feel it in your bones.

Seeing a loved one neglected naturally sparks anger. In the next chapter, we'll explore what to do with that anger when it seems no one is listening.

PATH POINTERS➤Neglected

Speak Up with a Script

Specific, kind, and time-bound get results.

Use: "I'm concerned about ___ because ___. Could we try ___ by ___ and review it on ___?"

Backup: invite a relative, trusted friend, or Parkinson's advocate to join in person or by speakerphone.

Build an Inside Ally

One staff member who "gets it" is gold.

How: learn names, thank specifically—"Thanks for cueing Mom's meds on time, it helped her eat"—and ask, "If I am worried, who should I contact first, and how?"

Document, Convene, Escalate

Logs turn anecdotes into action.

Track: date and time, who was present, what happened, what you requested.

Next: request a care conference and a short written plan with a review date. If issues continue, move up the chain (charge nurse → unit manager → director of care → patient relations or ombudsman). Ask about a Family Council.

Post the Essentials, Protect Your Stamina

Create a one-page "About Me" for the room: preferred foods, calming music, mobility cues, triggers, communication tips, and contact numbers.

After each visit: take five minutes to reset. Sit in the car, breathe, or text your ally an update so you can keep showing up.

Vary Your Visit Times

A different hour shows a different picture.

Plan: drop in at morning care, evening meals, and one weekend slot. Note hygiene, hydration, glasses, and hearing aids, and whether meds were given on time.

Today: put two varied visit times on your calendar.

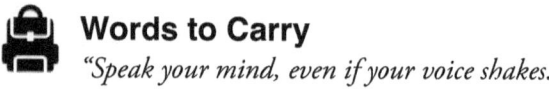 **Words to Carry**

"Speak your mind, even if your voice shakes."

—*Maggie Kuhn*

Angry (Part II)

ANGER MAKES ME UNCOMFORTABLE. I didn't want to write one chapter about it, let alone two. But Parkinson's brought anger more often than I expected, so here we are.

At first, I saw it in Mom more than in me. Over time, I couldn't avoid it either.

It hit when I realized I couldn't afford the care she needed. I remember thinking, *Lianna, you're in your late thirties and can't even keep the cottage or pay for full-time help. You've failed her.* Money became the villain in my head: If there had been more of it, maybe we could have kept the cottage; maybe Mom could have stayed out of long-term care.

Looking back, I also resented Mom a little for not being more financially prepared. I know that blame wasn't fair, but it was there—part grief over the cottage, part frustration watching PD derail the life she loved, part disappointment in facilities that couldn't meet her needs. Mostly, it was the disease.

Then our friend Carrie, whom we'd hired to add extra support at The Pines, told me there had been serious incidents on night shifts, including one fatality. She wasn't dramatic; she was matter-of-fact. If things didn't improve, the government might step in. My anger shifted from the abstract to the people in charge.

Hospital care was the next blow. Mom cracked her skull and needed seventeen stitches. They found her on the floor by the bathroom. In the ER, I asked what happened. "She hit a door frame," the nurse said. When I later asked about her Parkinson's meds—timing matters—the nurse looked blank and said she'd check. That's when anger and guilt hit at once. She had likely missed one or two doses.

"I'm so sorry, Mom," I whispered. I knew it wasn't my fault, but it felt like a failure.

In that moment, I realized something important: I was the expert in the room. Too many professionals didn't know that PD meds must be on time. That realization lit a fire. I became an advocate not just for Mom, but for anyone with Parkinson's.

Back at The Pines, I still couldn't relax. The same knowledge gaps were there. I promised myself: No more hospital visits becoming worse than they needed to be.

If you're navigating PD, don't assume hospital staff are trained in it. Go in prepared. The Parkinson's Foundation's Hospital Safety Guide is worth having in your bag. Facilities need the basics, too.

A few weeks after Mom returned, a thought I'd been pushing away surfaced: *Is this the beginning of the end?* I was stepping into grief deeper than anything I'd known.

That's where we'll go next—what grief felt like, and how I learned that loss isn't only about what's taken, but about what's left to carry.

PATH POINTERS ≻ Angry (Part II)

Name the Grief Under the Anger

Anger often covers loss or fear. When heat rises, ask: *What am I losing or protecting right now?*

Try now: say one line aloud: "Under this anger is ____." Then take one slow breath before you act.

Advocate with Tools

Go in prepared for hospital or facility visits.

Pack this: Parkinson's Foundation Hospital Safety Guide (med timing, communication notes). Outside the U.S., add Parkinson's UK Emergency Management of Patients with Parkinson's quick guide. One page on hand can change care.

Today: save both as PDFs on your phone and print a copy for your go-bag

Move It Through, Not at Someone

Give the surge a safe outlet so it does not land on people you love.

Options: a ten-minute "anger lap" outside, wall push-ups to light fatigue, or a song-length march in place.

Cue: stop when your breathing feels even.

Say It Early, Say It Clean

Short, specific statements prevent blowups.

Script starter: "I'm frustrated because ____ affects ____'s safety. I'm asking for ____. When can we review it?"

Facility add-on: "Who owns this, and what is the check-in date?"

See the Person; Blame the Disease

PD can skew mood and thinking. Hold the relationship while you address the symptom.

Set a reset: agree on a neutral pause word (for example, "reset"). When either person says it, both take sixty seconds, then return with one request and one offer.

Words to Carry

"I sat with my anger long enough until she told me her real name was grief."

Grief

I DEVOTED AN EARLIER CHAPTER to sadness, but grief goes deeper. As Parkinson's—and later dementia—chipped away at Mom, sadness settled into something rawer and more enduring.

I hesitated to write about grief. I don't want to imply everyone follows my mom's path or that her life with Parkinson's was only sorrow. It wasn't. But as the illness progressed, sadness became a steady companion. Tears came more often.

One evening at The Pines, our caregiver called to say Mom had had a rough day. When I arrived, she lay awake, eyes darting, low moans telling me she was scared. Was it sundowning, a medication effect, or both? I didn't know. I took her hand and whispered, "Mom, it's Lianna." She glanced at me and reached for the blanket at her waist. I tucked her in the way she once tucked me in.

It wasn't enough. Her agitation rose. Words tumbled out in a rush I couldn't catch, like a plea I couldn't translate. What I heard was the ache of dementia. What I saw was a woman trapped in a body that could no longer give her the life she deserved.

Fighting tears, I whispered, "It's okay if you're ready to go, Mom." I loved her too much to ask her to endure for me. In that moment, I let go.

I sat beside her until she finally slept. Walking out to the parking lot, I felt hollow. My aunt once told me it would get easier. I'm not sure it did; I think I just learned to carry the weight.

Looking back, I can see how I moved through grief in fits and starts. Not in neat order, but in loops:

- Denial: Telling myself things were better than they were to keep despair at bay.

- Anger: Plenty of it, as the earlier chapters show.

- Bargaining: The "if onlys"—more resources, different choices—maybe I could have spared her pain.

- Depression: Numbing with food, distraction, and unhelpful relationships when the load felt too heavy.

- Acceptance: Not of losing her, but of guiding her toward as much peace and comfort as possible.

Grief doesn't vanish, but with time and intention, its grip can loosen enough that you can breathe again.

It took us two and a half years to admit Mom needed a different home. We began the final move to a long-term care home where she was treated with genuine care. She felt seen there, and so did we.

That sense of being seen—of being respected and included—matters. Next, let's talk about feeling valued.

PATH POINTERS≻Grief

Let It Through

Grief moves when it's felt. Tears, anger, numbness—none of it is wrong.

Try this: set a ten-minute "grief window." Sit somewhere safe, name what hurts, and let the feeling rise and fall. When time ends, wash your face or step outside. Crying is one way we begin again.

Feel It With Music

Music can be a bridge to what's inside.

Build a two-track ritual: one song to open the feeling, like "Angels Among Us" (Alabama), and one to settle, like "Breathtaker" (SYML). Save a "Feelings" playlist for writing or release.

Borrow a Story

Books and films can hand you language (and company) when words are hard to come by.

Pick one:

> *The Year of Magical Thinking* by Joan Didion
>
> *A Grief Observed* by C.S. Lewis

A simple cue helps, like Sam's character in *Sleepless in Seattle* says, "I'm gonna get out of bed every morning and breathe in and out …" Sometimes routine is the first raft.

Plan the Tender Days

Anniversaries and firsts can sting.

Make a simple plan: choose a small ritual (light a candle, share a favorite photo, eat their go-to dessert) and text one person: "Heavy day this week—could we talk?"

Keep a Bond

Connection does not end; it changes.

Practice: write a short note to the person you miss, place a memento on a "memory shelf," or take a walk where you used to go together. Let warmth sit beside the ache.

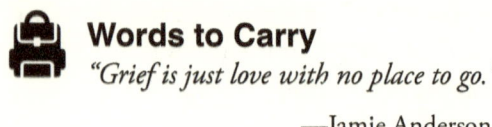 **Words to Carry**
"Grief is just love with no place to go."

—Jamie Anderson

Valued

I T TOOK FOUR NURSING HOMES to find the right fit. Looking back, there's plenty I would do differently if I'd understood long-term care better. But like so much of Mom's Parkinson's journey, we did the best we could with what we knew.

Mom spent her final two and a half years in a nursing home in Sudbury, Ontario—her birthplace. My aunt recommended it after her mother-in-law had a good experience there, and we were hopeful. It wasn't fancy, but genuine care made it stand out.

We need more staff who truly understand Parkinson's. Even one or two PD-savvy people in each home would change the daily lives of residents who don't fit the typical profile.

One practice I loved was the "Life Picture"—a collage of photos and short captions about each resident. Staff interviewed families (me, in Mom's case), gathered stories, and created a visual timeline that hung on the wall. It wasn't a small thing. It gave caregivers an instant way in: "You enjoy knitting, Val?" "Seven grandchildren—that must keep you busy!" It reminded everyone that this woman had lived a full life.

Other moments told us we mattered too:

- They welcomed a family piano so residents could enjoy music.

- Short-staffed or not, they took time to talk with us and listen.

- After Mom passed, they held an Honor Walk, staff lining the hall in silence.

- They invited us to a memorial service for residents who had passed that year.

These may not seem significant, but they meant everything. They said Mom wasn't "just another patient." She was known. I could leave visits feeling more at peace.

If you feel overlooked—whether you're living with Parkinson's or supporting someone who is—remember this: You deserve to be seen at every stage. You are not your diagnosis. And care partners, you are more than the invisible glue holding things together. Your worth doesn't fade when the road gets rough.

Whether it's a nurse who truly listens or a quiet hallway filled with respect, these moments are powerful. They say what we all need to hear: You matter. Our work is to believe it, and to treat ourselves with the same kindness we offer others.

Let's turn to what holds us when everything else feels uncertain: love.

PATH POINTERS➢Valued

Name Your Worth
Ask two trusted people to share one specific thing they value about you—and give one back in return. Save their words where you'll see them.

Today: text: "Quick favor: What's one thing you've valued in me lately? I'm collecting reminders."

Advocate Where You Are
Awareness grows when you lend your voice, whether in a care meeting or with a group like PD Avengers.

Try this: use a "thank-you + ask" script: "Thank you for ___; it helped. Could we also ___ for [name]?"

Check the Care Fit
If the current setup isn't serving your loved one, review and adjust. Small changes now prevent bigger problems later.

This week: "Walk the week." For seven days, note meals, meds, mood, and mobility. Then request a fifteen-minute care-plan huddle.

Give Back, Grow Roots
Service reinforces that you—and your story—matter. Volunteer, mentor, or join a fundraiser: a local walk, Team Fox, Pancakes for Parkinson's, Putts for PD, or Pickleball for a Purpose.

This month: pick one way to give back and put it on the calendar.

Practice Loving Boundaries
Love includes limits that protect everyone's energy. Saying no kindly keeps relationships strong.

Pocket lines: "I wish I could do that today. I can do ___ on ___." "I can stay for thirty minutes."

Today: choose one boundary you'll honor this week and tell one supportive person.

Explore Research, Eyes Open

Clinical trials can advance science and sometimes expand options.

Next step: ask your neurologist about current studies and review a plain-language consent together. Jot down pros and cons and your top three questions before deciding.

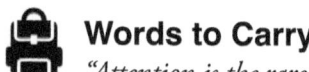 **Words to Carry**
"Attention is the rarest and purest form of generosity."

—Simone Weil

Loved

THEY SAY NO ONE LOVES YOU like your mom. For me, that was true. Mom's love was steady and generous, carrying me through every hard season. She cheered loudest, listened closely, and showed up. Not everyone gets that bond. I know how lucky I am.

Church was part of our Sundays growing up. I don't remember many sermons, but I loved "Children's Time," when Reverend Jerry, accordion in hand, told stories and sang just for us. One song, "The Magic Penny," stuck: Love grows the more you give it away.

Mom lived that lesson. Even after her Parkinson's diagnosis, she kept giving—starting a support group, showing up at fundraising walks, co-founding an organization for families like ours, and weaving love into the lives of her kids and grandkids. Her circle of care widened, not narrowed.

Love still showed up at home, too, but Parkinson's made it tricky for Mom and Dave. In the years when they still lived together, their roles had already shifted. Some days, it felt like care tasks crowded out everything else. They stumbled but made adjustments.

When dyskinesia made eating out difficult, they turned dinners into car picnics by the lake. When words would not come easily, they sat with hands touching and hummed along to Anne Murray songs. They kept small rituals: a funny show on TV in the evening, a short drive to look at the water, or a prayer before bed. There were hard moments. They might snap or go quiet, then come back to say sorry and make it right.

As the disease advanced, Dave learned transfers, medication timing, and how to read Mom's OFF periods. Mom learned to ask for help and to protect his rest. Love flowed both ways. That mattered.

Later, when they decided to live apart, and Mom moved into long-term care, Dave stayed faithful. He visited, advocated, and did the best he could for her.

For many couples, PD strains intimacy and identity. What helped Mom and Dave can help others: Name what is changing, keep talking even when it is awkward, and look for new ways to be close. Face Parkinson's as a shared challenge, not a solo battle.

If you're caring for a spouse or partner, protecting your own health and joy isn't selfish; it's essential. Strong couples are partners first, care partners second. When you're nourished, love has room to breathe.

Parkinson's does not erase love, intimacy, or partnership. It asks you to be creative, patient, and present in new ways. Joy and connection do not disappear. They evolve.

As we move forward, the next chapter—Blessed—looks at the quiet gifts that remain, and how noticing them can steady you for the road ahead.

PATH POINTERS➤Loved

Share One True Thing

Opening up builds connection and reminds you that you are not alone.

Today: tell one honest moment from your journey to someone safe (friend, group, or a short voice note). Keep it to five to ten sentences.

Boundary tip: if you do not want advice, add, "I'm sharing, not looking for fixes."

Love Yourself, Too

Caring for you is part of caring for your people.

This week: choose one small act of kindness for yourself each day—tea outside, a short podcast walk, or gentle stretches.

Make it real: add a daily calendar reminder titled "Care for me: ten minutes."

Protect the 'Us'

You are more than a patient and caregiver. Guard a pocket of time that belongs to both of you.

Try this: set a fifteen-minute ritual with no PD talk. Share a song, sit close, pray, or dream out loud.

If words are hard: ask plainly, "Could I have a hug?"

Name What Is Still Possible

Shift attention from limits to options.

Right now: finish this together: "Today we can ___." Do that one thing, then mark it with a small celebration.

Make Daily Deposits

Feed the bond with the Three T's.

- **Touch:** hold hands, a shoulder squeeze, or a thirty-second hand massage
- **Time:** a standing coffee, a sunset sit, a shared show
- **Talk:** one memory, one joke, one hope

Pick two to deposit today.

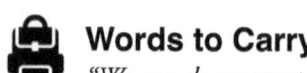 ## Words to Carry

"We can do no great things; only small things with great love."

—Mother Teresa

Blessed

WRITING MOM'S EULOGY CAME FASTER than I expected. I knew the day would come, but I hadn't paused to plan what I would say. I'm a writer, and I loved my mom. I did my best, but afterward I kept thinking of lines I wish I'd added.

I wish I'd told her how deeply I saw her daily struggle. Our routines filled every hour; then the battle ended. We were grateful, but we still lost Mom.

As I drafted my goodbye, I kept circling back to what she left behind. Among her few belongings were shoeboxes of photos—family, the lake, the cottage. Her friends were salt of the earth. That she had such loyal people in her corner says everything about her.

She also left us, her four kids. My younger sister and brother (and my older sister, who's no longer with us) are gifts I don't take for granted. Family was everything. In hard seasons, Mom leaned on her sister the way I leaned on mine. I'm blessed to call my siblings my closest friends.

Since we said goodbye, I've come to see the blessings that threaded through those many years with Parkinson's.

Not everyone likes the word *blessed*. Some prefer *lucky*. For me, *blessed* acknowledges the role faith played in our journey.

I believe Mom's life with Parkinson's was better because of her faith. Her relationship with God gave her purpose, strength, and a way to weather each day.

Her faith taught me to look for silver linings. Even as dementia crept in, her wit could spark in the dark. Smiles, hugs, and "I love you" gave us reasons to keep going. Sometimes she hummed "The Garden," the hymn she sang with her dad. When music cut through the fog and brought her back to us, it felt like a gift.

If she could speak for herself, I think she'd say she was blessed:

- to live longer than many with PD,

- to live a rich, full life,

- to be cared for by deeply kind people,

- to have a close, loving family.

As for me, the blessing has been the people I've met. Watching everyday tasks like tying shoes and brushing teeth turn into hard-won victories resets my perspective. People with Parkinson's hold on, keep going, and show a courage I'm humbled to witness.

I wouldn't wish PD on anyone, but living through Mom's journey changed me. I'm more patient, more empathetic, more present. Slowing down helped me see what matters, even when that was hardest to do.

In the end, I'm sure God was with us, even when I couldn't see it. I often picture "Footprints in the Sand": two sets on the beach, then one in the hardest stretches. The promise is simple—those were the moments you were carried. That image still steadies me.

Whether you believe in God, a higher power, or something else, I hope you can feel carried through your hard days with Parkinson's.

We're nearing the end of this journey together. Next, we'll sit with a destination I wish for all of us: peace.

PATH POINTERS≻Blessed

Expect Something Good
Train your attention to notice grace notes. Begin the day assuming at least one kindness will find you.

Today: name one small thing you are looking forward to and put it on a sticky where you will see it.

Name the Blessing
When something kind lands, pause and mark it. Gratitude grows when it is spoken.

Try this: whisper "thank you," send a one-line appreciation text, or add a tally mark to a "Blessings" note on the fridge.

Keep a Simple Daily Reading
If faith steadies you, choose a one-page devotional. If not, pick a brief reflective piece, such as a reader or a poem. One page is enough.

Cue: keep the book by the kettle or coffee maker and read while it heats.

Soundtrack Your Gratitude
Music can tilt your lens toward blessing. Build a "Blessed" mini-playlist with three to five songs.

Starter adds: "Count Your Blessings" (Johnson Oatman), "Blessed" (Martina McBride), "Blessings" (Laura Story).

Today: add one song and save the playlist to your home screen.

Remember, You Are Still Here
Presence is a blessing. Hand on heart: "I am still here; there is still good I can do today."

If faith language fits: "If you are not dead, God is not done."

If not: "As long as I am here, purpose remains."

Now: take one small step that matches that purpose.

 Words to Carry

"How lucky I am to have something that makes saying goodbye so hard."

—Winnie the Pooh

Peaceful

MOM PASSED AWAY QUIETLY on a Tuesday morning in January. After a brief bout of pneumonia, her heart finally rested. She spent her last days sleeping peacefully at the nursing home, my aunt holding her hand until the end. I find comfort knowing she wasn't alone.

Her death certificate lists "natural causes," but we know it was the thirty-year weight of Parkinson's and dementia that asked her body to say, "Enough."

Freed from relentless illness, Mom found peace.

Letting her go in her final days wasn't easy. I couldn't control Mom's passing any more than I could stop the slow erosion Parkinson's inflicted. Still, I prayed she wouldn't suffer.

Some people see long-term care as giving up. I don't. Accepting what we cannot change isn't surrender. We always sought the best care, but I learned there's only so much we can control.

Death ends our earthly journey; it is not failure. In the end, I'm at peace knowing we did what we could.

Watching Mom's last days made me think about life and legacy. Do memories matter if illness or time erases them? I believe they do. Loss reminds us that everything is temporary. That's life.

Chaucer wrote, "All good things must come to an end." I'd add: The hard things end, too. Suffering doesn't last forever.

After thirty years with a debilitating disease, her story deserves the truth. Honoring her means telling the whole story—the pain and despair, and the good that kept breaking through: music, laughter, ordinary mercies.

Parkinson's brought shock, frustration, and fear. It embarrassed us, left us neglected at times, and sometimes made us feel utterly lost. And still, we discovered comfort, connection, strength, and resilience. We found creativity and perspective. We learned to treasure simple joys—even in the midst of Parkinson's.

Mom is gone, but her legacy endures—in these pages, in the All About Parkinson's community, and in the memories she gave us. Writing this book has shown me how those years shaped me; the emotions have deepened my life, shifted my perspective, and given it purpose.

I hope never to face this disease myself. If I do, I trust Mom prepared me well.

As you walk your own path, may you see challenges not as stopping points but as invitations to discover your inner strength. Meet each moment with courage and grace, knowing you are not alone on the Parkinson's path.

Keep moving forward with determination, and may your days hold peace, meaning, and the hope that carries us through.

PATH POINTERS➤Peaceful

Let Go Boldly
Release what keeps you stuck. Create a tiny "release" ritual: Write one fear on a scrap of paper, read it once, then tear it and toss it. Repeat weekly.

Be Patient with Yourself
Peace unfolds on its own clock. Choose a gentler phrase for rough days—"I'm healing on time"—and stick it on your mirror.

Pause and Reframe
When you catch a heavy thought, zoom out (*What really matters here?*), then zoom in (*What's one kind thing I can do next?*). Your outlook shapes your outcome.

Rediscover Wonder
Let your inner kid lead for an hour: Rewatch a childhood favorite (*Hook*), build something simple, or stargaze. Wonder softens edges.

Engage with Purpose
Meaning rarely arrives by accident. Volunteer once, record one story, or start a small "legacy" project. Circle one doable step this month and schedule it.

Let Music Speak
Some feelings only songs can carry. Start a two-track "peace" pair:

- "Til You're Home" (Rita Wilson)
- "The Dance" (Garth Brooks)

Play them when you need a steadier breath.

Seek Wisdom in Pages

Pick one perspective-shifting read and browse a single chapter tonight:

- *The Awakened Brain* by Lisa Miller, on the science of spirituality and resilience
- *Ikigai* by García and Miralles, on small daily meaning and long-term joy.

Savor Small Moments

Slow the day on purpose: Sip something warm on the porch, notice one scent, one color, one kind face. Name them out loud.

Live Fully by Giving

Giving is living. Offer one small gift this week—time, attention, a note, a ride. Acts of service settle the heart.

Share Your Gifts

Your story lights paths. Tell one honest paragraph (to a friend, journal, or support group) and end with, "Here's what helped."

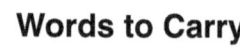 ## Words to Carry

"You have peace," the old woman said, "when you make it with yourself."

—Mitch Albom, The Five People You Meet in Heaven

When Other Feelings Show Up

NOT EVERY EMOTION FITS NEATLY into a single chapter. Some arrive quietly, then linger in the background: feelings like guilt, jealousy, overwhelm, and even relief. These emotions can surprise us, showing up alongside love, strength, or grief, often when we least expect them.

You may not talk about them often, but they're real, and they matter. They're part of what it means to be human while navigating Parkinson's—whether you live with it or care for someone who does.

What follows are a few reflections on these quieter companions: what they taught me, and what they might reveal to you.

Guilty

I felt guilty for so many things. Not that anyone can plan a life around having a mom with Parkinson's, but there were moments I didn't handle well, and things I wish I'd done differently. The good thing about guilt is that it pushed me to do better next time.

I don't know if Mom felt guilt herself. Knowing her, she may have carried a little for being "a burden" to her kids, though she never said it out loud. If she had, I would have stopped her right there.

In her later years, guilt showed up for me in new ways. When I caught myself feeling happy—really happy—I'd think, *How can I be happy, when she isn't?* It took time to see that joy wasn't betrayal. Both could exist at once: her struggle and my moments of lightness.

Guilt often points to love twisted into self-blame. It means we care. Sometimes too much. The work is to let that care guide us, not punish us.

Try this: When guilt rises, ask, *Did I truly do something wrong, or am I just feeling human?* If it's the latter, take a slow breath and let that be enough.

Jealous

I don't blame her for feeling jealous. Watching her body slowly lose control, how could she *not* envy every non-disabled person she saw? She wouldn't have been human if she didn't.

Sometimes Mom felt jealous that Dave got breaks from caregiving—time away at his support group, free from the constant demands of Parkinson's. "Why does *he* get time off Parkinson's when I don't?" she asked me once. I didn't have an answer. I'd never thought of it that way before.

I felt jealousy too—of friends with what I call "PPs," perfect parents. The ones who were not only still alive, but also healthy. Some even happily married. I envied peers who could chase new dreams without guilt, who didn't have to weigh every choice against someone else's growing needs.

Jealousy is a hard feeling to admit, but it's a mirror more than a flaw. It points to what we long for, what we've lost, or what we wish could be easier. When we name it without shame, it softens—and sometimes even shows us what matters most.

Try this: When envy stirs, ask gently, *What does this feeling want me to notice or protect?* Then take one small step toward that need.

Overwhelmed

There is so much to Parkinson's; no one could ever fit it all into one book. If you haven't felt overwhelmed at some point in this journey—whether you live with the disease or care for someone who does—you might be one of the rare few.

Many people describe feeling overwhelmed even before diagnosis. They knew something was wrong, but couldn't name it yet. Simple tasks like writing an email or following a recipe started taking hours instead of minutes because their thinking had changed. Confusion, fatigue, and frustration built long before the words *"You have Parkinson's"* were spoken.

Writing this book has reminded me of that same feeling. At times, it was overwhelming—wanting to get it right, to balance honesty with hope, to serve you, the reader, in a way that feels true.

Overwhelm comes when too much arrives at once. The brain can't sort or pace it, so everything feels urgent. In those moments, zoom in. One thing at a time. One breath, one task, one next right step.

I know how cliché this sounds, but "one day at a time" still works. And for Parkinson's, sometimes it's one *minute* at a time. Prioritize. Say no when you need to. Remind yourself—and others—that you're not superhuman. You don't have to do everything to be enough.

Try this: When everything feels like too much, pause. Say out loud, *"Right now, I'll do this one thing."* Then do only that.

Relieved

I hate using the word *relieved* when I talk about my mom's passing. But I was. Not because I wanted her gone, but because she was finally free from the struggle. The years of strain on her body, the hallucinations, the fear, the unrelenting fatigue—gone. That relief came with its own kind of guilt, but underneath it was love. I didn't want her to suffer anymore.

Many care partners feel this, though few admit it out loud. Relief after a loved one's death can feel like betrayal, but it isn't. It's a natural release after years of vigilance and worry. You've carried so much for so long that when the load lifts, your body and heart don't quite know what to do. Relief is the nervous system catching up to peace.

People with Parkinson's sometimes feel relief, too—though it shows up differently. Some have told me that getting a diagnosis, after months or years of unexplained symptoms, brought relief because it gave them a name for what was happening. Others feel moments of relief after a medication adjustment, a calm day, or finally accepting help. It's that quiet exhale that says, *I can rest for a moment.*

Relief doesn't cancel grief. It sits beside it. You can feel both at once: gratitude that suffering has ended and sorrow that a chapter has closed.

Try this: If you feel relief, let it come. You don't need to justify it. Whisper, *"It's okay to rest now."* Then take one deep, steadying breath—for both of you.

Before You Go

If Your Feeling Isn't in This Book

No book could name every emotion that surfaces along the Parkinson's path. Some will appear quietly; others will surge and surprise you. Whatever shows up, it's yours—and it's valid.

If your feeling isn't in these pages, try meeting it with curiosity and kindness:

- **Name it.** Give it a simple label: *I feel cheated, I feel envious.*

- **Normalize it.** Remind yourself: *Someone else on this path has felt this, too.*

- **Notice the story.** Ask: *What is my mind telling me about this feeling?*

- **Narrow it.** Choose one small action that would help today, not forever.

- **Nurture yourself.** Do one kind thing for your body or heart before the day is over.

There's no single way to feel—or heal—when living with Parkinson's. Every emotion, even the messy ones, is part of being human. Keep naming what's real, keep softening toward yourself, and keep walking your path with as much grace as you can.

 Final Words to Carry
"As you start to walk on the way, the way appears."

—Rumi

Acknowledgements

Thank you, reader. When I first began writing to the All About Parkinson's community in 2005, I never imagined that what started as a small effort to support my mom would grow into a global conversation that has lasted for more than twenty years.

Whether you're reading from Australia, Canada, France, Germany, Ireland, Mexico, New Zealand, Spain, the UK, or the US—and from countless other corners of the globe—it has been one of the great honors of my life to walk this path with you. Your stories, your courage, and your willingness to share your own journeys have shaped mine in ways I could never have expected.

Thank you, Mom, for encouraging me to write and for inspiring me to keep moving forward, no matter what challenges appeared along the way. You will always be my "why" for the work I do with the Parkinson's community and the heart behind every page of this book. And thank you, Dave, for caring for Mom with such devotion and for doing your best to navigate Parkinson's without a map. Your courage and commitment shaped the path we all walked together.

I can't thank my husband, Nick, enough for loving and supporting me through life's ups and downs, and for patiently enduring my endless overanalyzing throughout the writing process. Your steady belief in me—especially when I second-guessed myself—helped bring this book to life.

Thank you to my brother, Tim, and my sister, Tanya, for always lending an ear when I need one and for offering thoughtful feedback on my writing. And thank you to your wonderful kids, who bring me so much joy and are always willing to share their opinions on my book covers—they truly brighten the creative process.

I am grateful to be surrounded by a wonderful extended family, including my rockstar aunts Muriel, Susan, and Brenda, and my uncles Marty and Blaine. Each of you has been touched by Parkinson's in your own way, and your strength continues to inspire me. I hope this book honors both Mom's legacy and Uncle Brendon's, as well as the resilience our family has shown throughout the journey.

My sincere thanks to my good friend, Dr. Tim Ihrig. As a fellow writer and advocate for living well with illness, you inspire me to think more deeply, care more fully, and show up with greater intention. I'm grateful for our conversations and for the many life lessons you've shared along the way.

Thank you to Mark Warenycia for your continued tech support and marketing assistance at All About Parkinson's. Your generosity, expertise, and quiet dedication to this community have made an enormous difference. Your selfless commitment does not go unnoticed.

Thank you to the fantastic folks at the American Parkinson Disease Association. I am especially grateful to the APDA Northwest team, whose dedication and compassion embody what it means to truly show up for the PD community. Working alongside you is an honor, and I'm proud to be part of a team so committed to helping people live well with Parkinson's.

And above all, I'm grateful to God for the strength, peace, and guidance that sustained me throughout this journey.

About the Author

Lianna Marie is a best-selling author, speaker, and passionate advocate for the Parkinson's community. For thirty years, she served as caregiver and chief cheerleader for her mom, walking with her through every stage of the disease as they learned and adapted together.

Determined to make the journey easier for others, Lianna founded AllAboutParkinsons.com, an online hub that has connected tens of thousands of people with Parkinson's, their families, and caregivers worldwide. She currently serves as the American Parkinson Disease Association (APDA) Regional Director of Marketing and Communications, helping advance awareness, education, and support for those impacted by Parkinson's across multiple communities.

Her breakthrough handbook, *Everything You Need to Know About Parkinson's Disease*, has reached readers in nearly fifty countries and spent multiple weeks on Amazon's Parkinson's best-seller list. She followed it with *Everything You Need to Know About Caregiving for Parkinson's Disease* and *The Complete Guide for People with Parkinson's Disease and Their Loved Ones*, trusted resources praised for their clear language and heartfelt advice.

A former international medalist in modern pentathlon and swimming, Lianna competed for Canada before settling in the Pacific Northwest, where she now lives with her husband. When she isn't writing or speaking, you'll likely find her training laps in the pool—or answering reader questions at LiannaMarie.com.

A Note from the Author

If this book supported you in any way, I would be grateful if you'd consider leaving a brief review where you purchased it. Reviews help this book find its way to others who may be feeling overwhelmed or unsure—and I personally read every one. Your words truly matter.

Notes

Akeelah and the Bee, directed by Doug Atchison (2006; Los Angeles: Lionsgate, film).

Always Looking Up: The Adventures of an Incurable Optimist, by Michael J. Fox (New York: Hyperion, 2009).

The Anatomy of Hope: How People Prevail in the Face of Illness, by Jerome Groopman (New York: Random House, 2004).

"Angels Among Us," performed by Alabama (1993; RCA Nashville, digital audio).

Anger: Wisdom for Cooling the Flames, by Thich Nhat Hanh (New York: Riverhead Books, 2001).

Another Country: Navigating the Emotional Terrain of Our Elders, by Mary Pipher (New York: Riverhead Books, 1999).

The Art of Happiness: A Handbook for Living, by His Holiness the Dalai Lama and Howard C. Cutler (New York: Riverhead Books, 1998).

Atlas of the Heart: Mapping Meaningful Connection and the Language of Human Experience, by Brené Brown (New York: Random House, 2021).

The Awakened Brain: The New Science of Spirituality and Our Quest for an Inspired Life, by Lisa Miller (New York: Random House, 2021).

A Beautiful Day in the Neighborhood, directed by Marielle Heller (2019; Los Angeles: TriStar Pictures, film).

Beyond the Pale, performed by Jim Gaffigan (2006; New York: Comedy Central Records, DVD).

The Biggest Little Farm, directed by John Chester (2018; Los Angeles: Neon, film).

"Blessed," performed by Martina McBride (2001; RCA Nashville, digital audio).

"Blessings," performed by Laura Story (2011; Fair Trade Services, digital audio).

The Book of Joy: Lasting Happiness in a Changing World, by His Holiness the Dalai Lama and Archbishop Desmond Tutu, with Douglas Abrams (New York: Avery, 2016).

"Brave," performed by Sara Bareilles (2013; Epic Records, digital audio).

"Breathtaker," performed by SYML (2022; Nettwerk Music Group, digital audio).

The Bucket List, directed by Rob Reiner (2007; Los Angeles: Warner Bros. Pictures, film).

Carol Burnett, comedy sketches.

Burnout: The Secret to Unlocking the Stress Cycle, by Emily Nagoski and Amelia Nagoski (New York: Ballantine Books, 2019).

"Carry On," performed by fun. (2012; Fueled by Ramen, digital audio).

The Comfort Book, by Matt Haig (New York: Penguin Life, 2021).

"Count Your Blessings," by Johnson Oatman Jr., 1897.

The Daily Stoic: 366 Meditations on Wisdom, Perseverance, and the Art of Living, by Ryan Holiday and Stephen Hanselman (New York: Portfolio/Penguin, 2016).

"The Dance," performed by Garth Brooks (1990; Capitol Nashville, digital audio).

The Dance of Anger: A Woman's Guide to Changing the Patterns of Intimate Relationships, by Harriet Lerner (New York: Harper & Row, 1985).

Daring Greatly: How the Courage to Be Vulnerable Transforms the Way We Live, Love, Parent, and Lead, by Brené Brown (New York: Gotham Books, 2012).

Deep Work: Rules for Focused Success in a Distracted World, by Cal Newport (New York: Grand Central Publishing, 2016).

"Don't Stop Believin'," performed by Journey (1981; Columbia Records, digital audio).

"Don't Stop Me Now," performed by Queen (1979; EMI Records, digital audio).

Karla Hildebrandt Kroeker, "Effect of Health on Self-Identity: An Autoethnography," *Journal of Sociology and Christianity* 12, no. 1 (Spring 2022).

Feel the Fear and Do It Anyway, by Susan Jeffers (New York: Ballantine Books, 1987).

Field of Dreams, directed by Phil Alden Robinson (1989; Universal City, CA: Universal Pictures, film).

"Fight Song," performed by Rachel Platten (2015; Columbia Records, digital audio).

The Five People You Meet in Heaven, by Mitch Albom (New York: Hyperion, 2003).

"Footprints in the Sand." Often attributed to Mary Stevenson (circa 1930s) and sometimes to Margaret Fishback Powers. Authorship disputed.

Get Out of Your Mind and Into Your Life: The New Acceptance and Commitment Therapy, by Steven C. Hayes and Spencer Smith (Oakland, CA: New Harbinger Publications, 2005).

The Gifts of Imperfection: Let Go of Who You Think You're Supposed to Be and Embrace Who You Are, by Brené Brown (Center City, MN: Hazelden Publishing, 2010).

A Grief Observed, by C. S. Lewis (San Francisco: HarperOne, 2001).

Groundhog Day, directed by Harold Ramis (1993; Los Angeles: Columbia Pictures, film).

Happier: Learn the Secrets to Daily Joy and Lasting Fulfillment, by Tal Ben-Shahar (New York: McGraw-Hill, 2007).

The Happiness Advantage: The Seven Principles of Positive Psychology That Fuel Success and Performance at Work, by Shawn Achor (New York: Crown Business, 2010).

"Happy," performed by Pharrell Williams (2013; Columbia Records, digital audio).

Judy Long, "Helplessness & Hope in Parkinson's," YouTube video, Davis Phinney Foundation for Parkinson's, published December 18, 2019.

"Here Comes the Sun," performed by The Beatles (1969; Apple Records, digital audio).

Hidden Figures, directed by Theodore Melfi (2016; Los Angeles: 20th Century Fox, film).

The Honest Guys, YouTube channel.

Hook, directed by Steven Spielberg (1991; Culver City, CA: TriStar Pictures, film).

Hope and Help for Your Nerves: End Anxiety Now, by Claire Weekes (New York: Berkley Books, 2020).

The How of Happiness: A Scientific Approach to Getting the Life You Want, by Sonja Lyubomirsky (New York: Penguin Press, 2008).

"How to Become More Grateful, and Why That Will Make You Happier, Healthier, and More Resilient," *Chasing Life*, by David G. Allan (CNN), published May 19, 2022, podcast audio.

The Hundred-Foot Journey, directed by Lasse Hallström (2014; Los Angeles: Walt Disney Studios Motion Pictures, film).

Ikigai: The Japanese Secret to a Long and Happy Life, by Héctor García and Francesc Miralles (New York: Penguin Books, 2017).

"I Love It," performed by Icona Pop featuring Charli XCX (2012; TEN Music Group/Big Beat Records, digital audio).

"I'm Still Standing," performed by Elton John (1983; Geffen Records, digital audio).

Inside Out, directed by Pete Docter (2015; Emeryville, CA: Pixar Animation Studios, film).

Inside Out 2, directed by Kelsey Mann (2024; Emeryville, CA: Pixar Animation Studios, film).

The Intouchables, directed by Olivier Nakache and Éric Toledano (2011; Paris: Gaumont, film).

I Thought It Was Just Me (But It Isn't): Making the Journey from "What Will People Think?" to "I Am Enough", by Brené Brown (New York: Gotham Books, 2007).

"It's a Great Day to Be Alive," performed by Travis Tritt (2000; Columbia Nashville, digital audio).

It's a Wonderful Life, directed by Frank Capra (1946; Los Angeles: RKO Radio Pictures, film).

"It's OK (Acoustic)," performed by Nightbirde (2021; Nightbirde Records, digital audio).

"I Will Survive," performed by Gloria Gaynor (1978; Polydor Records, digital audio).

Keeping Up Appearances, created by Roy Clarke (1990–1995; London: BBC Studios, television series).

"Lean on Me," performed by Bill Withers (1972; Sussex Records, digital audio).

The Let Them Theory: A Life-Changing Tool That Millions of People Can't Stop Talking About, by Mel Robbins (Audible Studios, 2024), audiobook.

"Lonely People," performed by America (1974; Warner Bros. Records, digital audio).

Man's Search for Meaning, by Viktor E. Frankl (Boston: Beacon Press, 2006).

Marcel the Shell with Shoes On, directed by Dean Fleischer Camp (2021; Los Angeles: A24, film).

Dr. Bradley McDaniels, Karl Robb, and Angela Robb, "Quality of Life, Purpose, and Parkinson's Disease," YouTube video, published January 23, 2023.

My Little Ikigai Journal, by Amanda Kudo (New York: St. Martin's Griffin, 2018).

Nate Bargatze, stand-up comedy material (general reference).

The One Thing: The Surprisingly Simple Truth Behind Extraordinary Results, by Gary Keller and Jay Papasan (Austin, TX: Bard Press, 2013).

On Golden Pond, directed by Mark Rydell (1981; Beverly Hills, CA: Universal Pictures, film).

Paddington 2, directed by Paul King (2017; London: StudioCanal, film).

Patch Adams, directed by Tom Shadyac (1998; Universal City, CA: Universal Pictures, film).

The Peanut Butter Falcon, directed by Tyler Nilson and Michael Schwartz (2019; Los Angeles: Roadside Attractions, film).

Robert Plutchik, "Wheel of Emotions" model (general reference to psychological theory).

The Princess Bride, directed by Rob Reiner (1987; Los Angeles: 20th Century Fox, film).

"Rise Up," performed by Andra Day (2015; Warner Bros. Records, digital audio).

"Roar," performed by Katy Perry (2013; Capitol Records, digital audio).

Schitt's Creek, created by Eugene Levy and Daniel Levy (2015–2020; Toronto: Not a Real Company Productions/CBC Television/Pop TV, television series).

Seabiscuit, directed by Gary Ross (2003; Universal City, CA: Universal Pictures, film).

The Secret Life of Walter Mitty, directed by Ben Stiller (2013; Los Angeles: 20th Century Fox, film).

"Shake It Out," performed by Florence + The Machine (2011; Island Records, digital audio).

Singin' in the Rain, directed by Gene Kelly and Stanley Donen (1952; Beverly Hills, CA: Metro-Goldwyn-Mayer, film).

Sleepless in Seattle, directed by Nora Ephron (1993; Los Angeles: TriStar Pictures, film).

A Small Book About a Big Problem: Meditations on Anger, Patience, and Peace, by Edward T. Welch (Greensboro, NC: New Growth Press, 2017).

Soul, directed by Pete Docter (2020; Emeryville, CA: Pixar Animation Studios, film).

"The Sound of Silence," performed by Disturbed (2015; Reprise Records, digital audio).

"The Sound of Silence," performed by Simon & Garfunkel (1964; Columbia Records, digital audio).

STILL: A Michael J. Fox Movie, directed by Davis Guggenheim (2023; Los Angeles: Apple Original Films, film).

Stillness Is the Key, by Ryan Holiday (New York: Portfolio/Penguin, 2019).

The Theory of Everything, directed by James Marsh (2014; Los Angeles: Focus Features, film).

"Three Little Birds," performed by Bob Marley and the Wailers (1977; Island Records, digital audio).

"'Til You're Home," performed by Rita Wilson (2022; Decca Records, digital audio).

Traveling Mercies: Some Thoughts on Faith, by Anne Lamott (New York: Pantheon Books, 1999).

Tuesdays with Morrie: An Old Man, a Young Man, and Life's Greatest Lesson, by Mitch Albom (New York: Doubleday, 1997).

"Weightless," performed by Marconi Union (2011; Just Music, digital audio).

"What a Wonderful World," performed by Louis Armstrong (1967; ABC Records, digital audio).

When the Body Says No: Exploring the Stress-Disease Connection, by Gabor Maté (Hoboken, NJ: John Wiley & Sons, 2003).

When Things Fall Apart: Heart Advice for Difficult Times, by Pema Chödrön (Boston: Shambhala Publications, 1997).

Won't You Be My Neighbor?, directed by Morgan Neville (2018; Los Angeles: Focus Features, film).

The Year of Magical Thinking, by Joan Didion (New York: Alfred A. Knopf, 2005).

"You'll Never Walk Alone," performed by Josh Groban (2015; Reprise Records, digital audio).